THE HEALTH SCANDAL

*Your Health
in Crisis*

Vernon Coleman

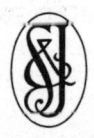

SIDGWICK & JACKSON LTD
LONDON

First published in Great Britain in 1988 by
Sidgwick & Jackson Limited

Copyright © 1988 by Vernon Coleman

ISBN 0-283-99509 2

Photoset by Rowland Phototypesetting Limited
Bury St Edmunds, Suffolk
Printed by Butler & Tanner Limited
Frome and London
for Sidgwick & Jackson Limited
1 Tavistock Chambers
Bloomsbury Way
London WC1A 2SG

TO TONY AND GERTRUDE

ACKNOWLEDGEMENTS

A full list of the people who have helped me with this book would take up so much space that there would be hardly any room left for the text. But special thanks are due to Tony Sharrock who nagged me into writing it, David Harsent, Jane Turnbull, Sue Ward and Susan Hill of Sidgwick and Jackson. I would also like to thank my readers for their letters of encouragement and support.

CONTENTS

PROLOGUE

The Future We Face

By the year 2020 one-third of the population in the developed world will be over the age of sixty-five. One-quarter of the population will be diabetic. In every home where there are two healthy parents and two healthy children there will be four disabled or dependent individuals needing constant care. Diseases such as diabetes and schizophrenia (which are genetically transmitted) and blindness (which is ten times as common among the over sixty-fives and thirty times as common among the over seventy-fives) will be as common as indigestion and hay fever are today. Unemployment will be normal. Stress-related diseases will be endemic. Developed countries around the world will face bankruptcy as they struggle to find the cash to pay pensions, sick pay and unemployment benefits.

Resentment, bitterness and anger will divide the young and the old, the able-bodied and the dependent, the employed and the unemployed. There will be anarchy, despair and civil war. There will be ghettoes of elderly and disabled citizens abandoned to care for themselves. There will be armed guards on our hospitals. Those with jobs will travel to work in armoured cars.

For years those who have forecast the end of the human race have talked of nuclear war, starvation in the third world, and pollution as being the major threats to our survival. But the decline I predict for the year 2020 will be triggered not by any of these forces but by much simpler and entirely predictable developments. The human race will be destroyed by medical ambition, commercial greed, and political opportunism.

In those last desperate years as our species destroys itself, attempts will be made to restore the balance. Euthanasia will be widely advocated. Politicians will call for parents to submit to genetic checks before being issued with breeding licences. Murder will be seen as a social service. But it will be too late. By the year 2020

1

there will be no chance for us to avoid the inevitable. The decline of our species will continue rapidly.

There is, I believe, just time for us to save ourselves from this holocaust. But we must act quickly and firmly. And many of the things we must do to save ourselves will be controversial and unpopular. Later in this book I will explain exactly what I think we need to do. But first I want to explain exactly how and why things have gone so badly wrong.

THE DECLINE OF THE SPECIES

At the start of the nineteenth century life expectancy was low and babies and infants often died young. At the start of the nineteenth century the infant mortality rate – the number of children dying within a year of their birth – is believed to have been about 250 per 1,000. By the year 1900 it was 150 per 1,000. Ten years later it was down to 100 per 1,000. A century earlier diseases such as smallpox, typhoid, cholera, and tuberculosis devastated whole communities. In 1838, the first year that full figures were kept, 16,268 people died of smallpox. In 1899 there were twenty deaths from smallpox.

By the end of the nineteenth century the position had changed dramatically. Life expectancy had improved enormously and babies stood a much better chance of living to childhood or even adulthood. Improvements in public health facilities, in housing regulations, in food supplies, and in agricultural policies had all helped to ensure that people had more to eat, better homes to live in, cleaner water to drink and so greater protection against disease and infection. Social advances had enabled us to conquer many of the diseases that had for centuries threatened whole nations.

By the start of the twentieth century the future looked bright. The drugs industry was just developing and surgical skills were being honed to new high standards. Anyone alive at the start of this century could have felt confident that the medical profession would bloom and that in the future people would lead longer and healthier lives. But it hasn't turned out quite like that. And to the outsider it is probably difficult to understand exactly what has gone wrong.

Certainly no one can complain that we haven't spent enough money on health care. Within the last twenty years more money has been spent on medical care and research than was spent in the whole of the rest of man's history on earth. Health care has become one of the world's largest and fastest-growing industries. Every year we spend a greater and greater percentage of our Gross National Product on the National Health Service. In the 1960s we spent four per cent of our GNP on the NHS. In 1985 we spent six per cent of our GNP on the NHS. During the lifetime of the 1983–7 Conservative

3

Government spending on the health service increased by twenty-six per cent in real terms with the total amount being spent on the NHS reaching £20 billion in 1988. And while the NHS has continued to demand and use more and more money, the private health sector has also continued to grow with millions of taxpayers prepared to pay twice for the privilege of having good, effective health care. But we have virtually nothing to show for all the effort and money that has been spent.

Medicine has become full of confusions and paradoxes. The expenditure on health care has rocketed but the figures show that people are now more likely to fall ill than they were a generation ago. In April 1987 the Health Promotion Research Trust published details of its 'Health and Lifestyle Survey' which involved over 9,000 adults. They concluded that about one in three people in Britain now say that they suffer from a long-standing illness or disability. A survey conducted in Bermondsey in the 1970s showed that ninety-five per cent of the population considered themselves to have been unwell in the fourteen days prior to questioning.

We now spend more than ever on medical research. But D. F. Horrobin, Director of the Endocrine Pathophysiological Laboratory, Clinical Research Institute, Montreal, Canada has pointed out that 'in the very few areas where advances have been made, the work was begun well before 1958'. We spend more than ever on health care but no one could argue that there is any less suffering in our society. Indeed, the figures show that the number of people committing suicide is increasing every year. In 1978 a total of 4,022 men and women killed themselves. By 1983 the annual death toll from suicide had reached 4,279. In 1984 it was 4,315. In 1985 it was 4,419. These figures, from the Office of Population Censuses and Surveys, show a steady, but continuing increase. In December 1986 psychiatrist Dr John Merrill, speaking at a meeting in Birmingham organized by the West Midlands Poisoning Unit, reported that attempted suicides among the elderly had more than doubled over the last two years. Finally, in addition to the increase in the number of successful suicide attempts, an increasing number of people now attempt suicide – each year well over 100,000 people try to kill themselves in Britain.

The number of doctors goes up. But the evidence shows that people are more dissatisfied with their doctors than ever before. There is a widely held opinion among those whose job it is to assess the benefits of health care that the net value of modern medicine may be negative – in other words that over-treatment, bad treatment and abuse of technology means that doctors do, on balance, more harm than good. During doctors' strikes in America and Israel the death

4

rate actually fell – indeed, any time there has ever been a doctors' strike the mortality rate has fallen dramatically (see also p. 212).

It is widely agreed that eighty per cent of patients visiting a doctor need no treatment. But it is also widely acknowledged that about eighty per cent of people visiting a doctor will be given treatment. Speaking at a seminar on 'Children's Health in the 80s' held at the Royal Society of Medicine in 1987 Dr Brent Taylor, Senior Lecturer and Honorary Consultant Paediatrician at St Mary's Hospital, said that cough suppressants should never be used, and that hundreds and hundreds of gallons of antihistamines and decongestants are poured down children's throats without a shred of evidence that they alter the natural history of the condition for which they are prescribed. He stressed the importance of avoiding prescribing antibiotics for any respiratory infection since more than ninety per cent are caused by a virus and get better on their own. In an April 1987 issue of the *Veterinary Record* Professor Richard Laccy, Head of the Department of Microbiology at Leeds University, made a strong attack on doctors' antibiotic-prescribing habits. He claimed that by using antibiotics in conditions where there is little indication for their use, such as upper respiratory tract infections, infective diarrhoea, varicose ulcers, and bed sores doctors are responsible for the development of antibiotic resistance in bacteria. Speaking at a symposium held at the Royal Society of Medicine in 1983 a Professor Lant reported that more than fifty per cent of antibiotics were either not indicated or prescribed inappropriately. My own researches suggest that in general practice antibiotics are needed by only about ten per cent of the patients who are given them. The overuse of antibiotics causes unnecessary allergy reactions, side effects, and sometimes serious complications.

Every year doctors write out tens of millions of prescriptions for drugs which are known to do more harm than good. The overuse of drugs is endemic and numerous doctors have confirmed that side effects are so common that one in every ten hospital beds is occupied by a patient who has been made ill by a doctor's treatment. For example, in 1986 Dr Gareth Beevers, a physician at the Dudley Road Hospital in Birmingham and a lecturer in medicine at Birmingham University, estimated that ten to fifteen per cent of patients are in hospital with drug-related problems.

It has been estimated that probably only one-quarter of all prescriptions are necessary. So many prescriptions for commonly used drugs – antibiotics, painkillers, antacids, cough medicines, sleeping tablets, tranquillizers, vitamins and so on – are unnecessary that I doubt if I am the only doctor to believe that three-quarters of all prescriptions signed by British doctors are unnecessary. Around eighty per cent of the people who go to see a doctor have nothing wrong with them that wouldn't get better with a good holiday, a win on the pools, or a little friendship and understanding. People want doctors they can talk to and trust. They want guidance, support, kindness, and caring. But they get drugs. They get more and more dangerous and painful investigations. And they get ever more inhuman treatment. The despair and disappointment have led millions to turn to alternative practitioners who may be incompetent charlatans but who are kindly and patient.

We spend about eighty per cent of our £20 billion a year NHS budget on building and running hospitals. Those new hospitals are stuffed with remarkably sophisticated machinery and staffed by endless rows of well-paid administrators. We have intensive care units, transplant units, and surgeons performing miracles of science every day. And yet waiting lists get longer and longer and hundreds of thousands die every year while waiting for essential treatment. In 1985 a survey published in *Nursing Mirror* showed that rats, mice and cockroaches are now commonly seen running around in the wards and operating theatres of British hospitals. We have new buildings, better facilities, and improved techniques, yet hospitals are constantly overcrowded with thousands of patients having to sleep on temporary beds put up in the corridors. We have specialist coronary care units for heart-attack victims and more cardiologists than ever before. Heart transplantation is commonplace. And yet more people than ever are dying of heart disease. And a considerable amount of evidence shows that a man or woman who has a heart attack will be better off staying at home than going into hospital. In a review article published in *Update* in 1982, Dr Joseph H. Levenstein concluded that evidence from large surveys done by specialists in Bristol, Nottingham and Teeside had shown that very many heart-attack patients do just as well if they stay at home as they do if they go into hospital.

Doctors are paid better than ever before but their education is paid for largely by drug companies which finance meetings and medical journals. In a paper entitled 'The Consultant's Role in Continuing Medical Education of General Practitioners: The Case of Rheumatology', published in the *British Medical Journal* in January 1987, Elizabeth Badley and Jennifer Lee of the Arthritis and Rheumatism Council Epidemiology Research Unit at Manchester University concluded that 'the overall level of drug-company sponsorship is considerable'.

Prince Sadruddin Aga Khan, addressing the Medical Society of the World Health Organization, while consultant to the Secretary-General of the United Nations, pointed out that in Great Britain today half the adult population and a third of children take some form of medication every day.

We have conquered terror diseases such as polio and diphtheria, but one in six girls and one in nine boys will need to spend some time in a mental institution. Diseases of nature have been replaced by diseases of civilization such as those produced by pollution and stress. We lead the world in some esoteric areas of medical research and yet countless thousands of mentally-handicapped individuals roam the streets because we have no facilities for them. We give free sex-change operations to patients who want them, but we charge patients an inflated price for essential dental treatment, for spectacles, and for drugs they need to stay alive. In 1987, for example, the price of National Health Service prescription drugs went up nine per cent while the real cost of the drugs went up by 2.5 per cent. Many hundreds of products – antibiotics, antihistamines, painkillers, skin creams, indigestion remedies, and iron tablets, for example – cost less than the prescription charge.

We have been misled into thinking that we are healthier than our ancestors and that in health terms we have never had it so good. In fact the truth is very different.

The truth is that our society is becoming sicker and sicker every year. After reaching a peak a decade or more ago, for many life expectancy is now falling. Figures published by the United States Bureau of the Census show that thirty-three per cent of people born in 1907 could expect to live to the age of seventy-five whereas thirty-three per cent of the people born in 1977 could expect to live to the age of eighty. Hardly a great difference! Life expectancy has gone up little if at all. Many people are now living into their seventies, eighties and nineties, but there has been an increase in mortality rates among the middle-aged and an increase in the incidence of diseases such as heart disease, diabetes, arthritis, and other long-term disabling disorders. In 1975 figures published by the Central Statistical Office in London showed that a middle-aged man of forty-five could expect to live only four years longer than his grandfather. The British were never healthier than they were during the Second World War. The death rate of workmen over fifty years of age was higher in the 1970s than it was in the 1930s.

It is undoubtedly true that if a patient today has a specific, and preferably rare disease and is treated accurately for that disease, he will benefit more than at any other time in history. But it is also true that if a patient does not have a specific and treatable disease, or if the doctor gets the diagnosis wrong, then the patient may well be worse off than at any other time in our history.

Britain is not the only country where all this is happening. In just

7

about every so-called 'developed' country in the world official morbidity figures tell the same story. The incidence of many of the most long-term, crippling diseases is increasing at a rapid rate.

We have, I believe, reached a crisis point. The evidence shows that by the time we reach the year 2020 it will be too late to do anything to prevent the inevitable holocaust. Our society will be so weakened and so divided that recovery will be impossible. The 1981 British census figures showed that one in every five members of the population is a pensioner. In 1987 a survey organized for *Saga* magazine showed that thirty-three per cent of all adults in the United Kingdom are over fifty-five years of age. My estimate, based not only on current figures but on forecasts made by such august bodies as the International Monetary Fund, is that by 2020 one-third of the population will have reached retirement age. And at least half of the remaining adults will be chronic invalids, requiring permanent care and attention. That means that every single healthy adult in the developed world will be working for at least two other people and will have the physical responsibility of caring for two other people, too.

The year 2020 is significant because I estimate that in that year the number of disabled and dependent individuals in the developed world will exceed the number of able-bodied individuals. If I am wrong, then I am more likely to have underestimated the rate at which we will reach this crisis point. It is unlikely to be later than 2020. If you feel sceptical and suspect that this is alarmist, then let me just remind you that today, on average, one-third of the population of any developed country has poor health which affects their ability to work or to look after themselves. In March 1987 the Chest, Heart and Stroke Association revealed that one half of the beds in NHS hospitals are occupied by patients suffering from some sort of stroke. The NHS is being suffocated by the growing number of elderly or disabled individuals in our communities.

If you think that none of this could happen in our ever-caring society, then look around you and think carefully. Already I believe that if you look hard you can see signs that the rift between the able-bodied and the disabled is widening. There is resentment and bitterness. The employed are beginning to object to supporting the unemployed. There is anger about the expenditure of money on performing surgery to save the lives of the congenitally deformed or the seriously injured. Already there have been calls for euthanasia to be legalized. Doctors have denied help to smokers suffering from bronchitis. Surgeons have refused to operate on the overweight. There have been protests about parents having children they cannot support or afford. The courts have given doctors permission to sterilize the mentally handicapped.

Drug addicts are being denied proper medical help. Patients who smoke and who develop arterial disease are also denied medical help. Kidney transplants are performed only on patients with jobs, families and prospects. There is already a lack of compassion for the elderly, the disabled and the sick. The tide against the weak and the frail is beginning to turn in our society. Old people and handicapped people are mugged on the streets. And resentment is growing against those who rely on social-security benefits. People are beginning to make it clear that they do not want the elderly and the disabled kept alive at all costs. The signs of dissatisfaction are all around us.

In the past threats to the survival of the human race have always come from outside. We have been threatened by infectious diseases. Or by starvation due to failing crops. Always we have been threatened by problems which we could counteract by encouraging our scientists, politicians and industrialists to work together and come up with a solution. When we were threatened by starvation new ways were found of harvesting food. And to protect us from future problems better agricultural techniques were developed. When we were threatened by infection, scientists came up with better sewage facilities, cleaner water, quarantine, vaccination, and antibiotics.

This time the difference is that it is our scientists, politicians and industrialists who have helped to produce the problems we face. The aims and aspirations of those who, a generation or two ago, would have been dedicated to eradicating disease have been distorted by personal ambitions, professional loyalties, and commercial forces. In the past the most powerful forces in any society have always combined to oppose any threats from outside. Today the most powerful forces in society – science and commerce – are conspiring to make things worse. Our medical scientists have not only failed to understand the enormity of the disaster in front of us, but they are daily making things worse. The most powerful forces in the world of industry are so preoccupied with making profits for today that they have failed to see that they are helping to ensure their own eventual destruction.

I have been studying this problem for nearly fourteen years and I am now convinced that time is rapidly running out. If we do not take drastic action soon, all the available evidence suggests that within thirty-five years or so civilization will end. More than half of the world's population will be too ill or too old to work or even to look after themselves. For the first time in history the size of the population needing care and attention will exceed the size of the population fit enough to do the work and do the looking after. The situation will get rapidly worse with each succeeding month.

There are, I believe, fourteen quite separate and specific explanations for the crisis in which we now find ourselves. Each of these is a scandal in itself. And only by understanding the individual nature of each will it be possible for us to avoid the holocaust I have forecast. So what follows is a description in some detail of the fourteen health scandals of the twentieth century.

SCANDAL No. 1

Distortion and Deceit

We spend more on health care than ever before. We ought to be healthier than ever. Some people claim that we are healthier than ever. But we're not. Official statistics show that life expectation has reached a plateau and that an increasing number of young people – men and women in their thirties and forties – are dying of heart disease, strokes and cancer. The number of deaths due to heart disease has more than doubled since the start of this century and figures published by the Office of Population Censuses and Surveys show that the number of heart-attack patients who are admitted to hospital has gone up every year recently (despite the fact that a growing number of GPs are now keeping heart-attack victims at home). In 1979 a total of 88,970 heart-attack patients were admitted to hospital. In 1980 the figure was 90,000. In 1981 it was 94,640. In 1982 it was 96,650. In 1983 it was 99,140. In 1984 it had grown to 102,720. And by 1985 it had reached 107,010. Of the 60,000 men who died of sudden heart attacks in 1985 nearly a third were of working age.

More than at any other time in our history we know what causes disease. We know the risk factors involved in the development of heart disease. And we know how eighty per cent of all cancers develop. Yet, despite this knowledge, mortality and morbidity rates remain high. I believe that one of the reasons why our health is not improving is because there are many organizations today which have a vested interest in producing – and maintaining – a sense of confusion and uncertainty. Politicians, doctors, journalists and public relations experts hired by large companies and pressure groups all have their reasons for distorting the truth and replacing the real facts with their own favourite brand of fiction.

AIDS

Early in 1987 ex-soldier Michael Coles, a forty-two-year-old father of two, picked up a shotgun, blasted his eighteen-year-old son in the back, killed his thirty-nine-year-old wife Margaret and then turned the shotgun on himself. The coroner recorded that Mrs Coles had been unlawfully killed and that her husband had committed suicide. Andrew, their eighteen-year-old son, survived.

Michael Coles took this dreadful step because he thought he had Aids. He decided to wipe out his family in case he had infected them. And he decided to kill himself to avoid the misery and suffering that he considered inevitable. In fact he didn't have Aids at all. He had flu. But, like millions of other perfectly ordinary, healthy individuals, he had been terrified out of his mind by the propaganda from which it has been quite impossible to escape in the last few years.

Michael Coles, like many others, was convinced that Aids threatens us all, and that it is a common, easily caught, inevitably lethal disease. He had believed what his government had told him, what he'd heard on television and what he'd read in the newspapers. The real tragedy is that he, like everyone else, had been conned.

Aids is, without a doubt, a nasty disease. But it is also a relatively uncommon disease. And it will probably stay that way. From the facts that are available it is clear that Aids is not going to be the disease that wipes out mankind. Before I substantiate this claim, and outline a few basic facts about the disease, here is a true anecdote that will, perhaps, help to make it clear why the public image of this disease is so horribly inaccurate.

In early 1987 I had a telephone call from a researcher for a TV company who told me that he was planning a documentary about Aids.

'What do you think about Aids?' he asked me.

I told him that I thought that Aids was a serious problem, but it was just one of many serious medical problems and the threat it posed had been exaggerated by some doctors, a lot of politicians and most journalists. The researcher was silent for a moment or two. I could tell by the silence that he was disappointed. It wasn't quite what he'd hoped to hear.

'We're planning a major documentary,' he said. 'We want to cover all the angles. Haven't you got anything new to say about Aids?'

'I don't think Aids is a plague that threatens mankind,' I insisted. 'I think it is a dangerous, infectious disease that currently affects a small number of people and that may, in the next few years, affect thousands more.'

I then pointed out that I believed that the evidence about Aids had been distorted and the facts exaggerated.

'We really wanted you to come on to the programme and talk about some of the problems likely to be produced by the disease,' persisted the researcher.

'I'm happy to come on to the programme and say that I think that the dangers posed by the disease have been exaggerated,' I told the researcher.

The researcher sighed. 'Quite a few doctors have said that to me. But it really isn't the sort of angle we're looking for.'

Very gently, I put down the telephone.

I didn't expect to hear from the researcher again and I didn't. His company produced a networked television programme about Aids that appeared on our screens a short time after that conversation. And I suspect that most of those who viewed it will have gone to bed believing that Aids is the greatest threat to mankind since the Black Death.

That isn't an isolated anecdote. I don't mean to imply that television company is worse than any other, but it illustrates the point I want to make, which is that the facts about Aids have been carefully selected to satisfy the public image of the disease (and to provide a good spiky story) rather than to relate the truth.

So now, let's get back to some facts. First, the number of heterosexuals suffering from the disease who have contracted Aids in Britain.

As I write this, in the autumn of 1987, new figures from the DHSS have just shown that eight heterosexuals have now contracted Aids in Britain. That isn't eight people in 1987. Or eight people in 1986. It is ever. By September 1987 just eight heterosexuals had ever contracted Aids in Britain.

Just to put things in perspective I should perhaps point out that in the last two years in Britain no less than thirty-six people have died while horse-riding. Perhaps, instead of spending millions trying to encourage heterosexuals to wear condoms the Government should have been spending its money trying to encourage horse-riders to wear hard hats.

Now let's examine the projected outcome for this disease in the next year or two. According to 'experts' speaking on behalf of the Government and the British Medical Association Aids is threatening to decimate the British population before the decade is out. (Incidentally, in March 1986 Dr Philip Welsby, Consultant Physician in communicable diseases at the City Hospital in Edinburgh, pointed out in the medical newspaper *GP* that 'there are more so-called experts on Aids giving authoritative talks than there are patients with Aids'.) Politicians and some 'medical experts' seem agreed that the incidence of the disease is increasing so rapidly that within a few years every family in the country will be affected by it. An official spokesman for the BMA has been widely quoted as forecasting that within five years 400 people a month will be dying of the disease. It

13

has been said that every family in the UK will be touched by Aids and one gloomy prognosticator has warned us that by the year 2000 we will all have the disease. Once again when the facts are examined it is clear that this claim is exaggerated.

It is certainly true that in the last few years the incidence of Aids has increased rapidly. But only through a relatively small section of the population. Two specific groups have been particularly at risk; syringe-sharing drug users and promiscuous homosexuals. These two groups are at risk because Aids is essentially a disease that is transmitted through the blood (rather than a sexually-transmitted disease) and both these groups enjoy practices which involve possible contamination through an exchange of blood.

Although the British Government's main Aids campaign has been directed at heterosexuals, the vast majority of the cases where the disease has been transmitted have involved individuals who have either experimented with intravenous drug-taking or who have had homosexual partners. Indeed, in the *Journal of the American Medical Association* published data showed clearly that the Government's campaign had been both inappropriate and exaggerated. According to the study, which involved more than 1,000 heterosexuals, homosexuals, and bisexuals the *only* sexual practice which was found likely to lead to contracting Aids was receptive anal intercourse. Another study, conducted by the Center for Disease Control in Atlanta, Georgia (which has conducted much of the most authoritative research in Aids in America and which, in 1981, published the first report on the disease), showed that on average homosexuals who contract Aids have had 1,100 sexual partners.

This evidence is significant because it shows that although the incidence of Aids has increased fairly rapidly in the past the number of people suffering from the disease in the future is unlikely to continue at the same rate. The incidence of Aids in our society will be limited largely by the number of promiscuous homosexual men who enjoy receptive anal intercourse. Blood transfusion is – even in America – a relatively minor cause of Aids. The disease is still a predominantly homosexual disease. Aids is spread by anal intercourse because this is the only sexual activity that commonly causes bleeding and Aids is, as I've already pointed out, a blood-borne disease.

When making projections for the future the Government has always assumed that Aids will continue to spread at the same rate as it has spread for the last year or two. But for that to happen we would need a population which matched in composition the population which has so far been affected by Aids. In fact, the evidence strongly suggests that the growth of Aids will slow down as soon as the larger part of the promiscuous homosexual population has been infected.

Aids is a nasty disease. It is a disease that needs to be taken seriously. But it is not a major threat. There are dozens of medical problems which deserve our concern more than Aids. And doctors, journalists, and politicians could do far more to preserve our health by concentrating on tobacco and alcohol addiction than on Aids.

So, why, you may ask, has the Aids threat been exaggerated? There are, I believe, a number of possible explanations. First, Aids is an attractive 'media' disease. People love being terrified. That is why horror movies and supernatural books do so well. Aware of this, television companies and other media moguls are constantly on the lookout for new scare stories. That television researcher whom I mentioned earlier wasn't the only person working in TV who wanted to build up the myths about Aids.

A short while ago we were all being frightened out of our minds by Legionnaire's Disease. Then there was Herpes. Radiation sickness and Chernobyl almost pushed Aids aside, but a killer disease that is transmitted sexually makes irresistible copy. It really is its link to sex that makes Aids such a popular media disease. That is what enables the puritans to tell us we've got what we deserve and to talk incessantly about the wrath of God. It also enables the less prurient to show condoms on television in the interests of education.

Secondly, Aids is now very big business. And it means money to a lot of people. If you think I'm being unduly cynical about this, just ask any stockbroker what effects the Aids scare had on international drug company share prices. Or ask a medical researcher how much easier he finds it to get funding for projects loosely associated with Aids. Or ask a local private screening clinic how well business has done in the wake of the Aids panic.

In April 1987 *Fortune*, the American business magazine, ran a special feature entitled 'Aids stocks worth the gamble' in which it reported some of the remarkable profits that had been associated with the Aids scare. So, for example, investors were reminded that shares in Wellcome, the British drug company which had produced an anti-Aids drug called AZT, had rocketed by 360 per cent in just twelve months.

Some industry analysts recommended Abbott Laboratories which was at the time believed to control over half the US market for Aids-related blood tests. In 1986 Abbott sold between $30 and $40 million worth of tests to detect exposure to the Aids virus. Experts advising *Fortune* readers predicted the annual demand for tests would bring the company hundreds of millions of dollars a year.

Another big drug company to benefit from the Aids scare was (almost inevitably perhaps) the ubiquitous Hoffmann–La Roche.

Hoffmann—La Roche shares were recommended (despite the fact that they cost an extraordinary $129,870 each) on the rather slight grounds that the company was about to get a licence to develop, manufacture and market a drug called ddC that was thought to have some potential against Aids.

But the best proof of the financial value of the Aids overkill comes, perhaps, from the fact that in the first three months of 1987 a portfolio of shares in companies offering Aids solutions rose by a magnificent forty-one per cent.

Finally, there is a third possible reason why Aids became so popular. And why it was for a while impossible to turn on a television set without seeing yet another Government-sponsored commercial telling us all of the dangers of this particular disease. Politics.

1987 was an election year. And it is difficult to avoid the conclusion that Aids was the 1987 equivalent of the Falklands War. Many political commentators believe that the war in the Falklands helped the Conservatives win the 1983 election. When the political climate is unsettled, when there are dangers threatening our very existence, and when the enemy is threatening and mysterious, we tend to turn for security to something that seems strong and powerful. We vote for the strongest party. Is it possible, I wonder, that Conservative politicians could have built the Aids scare into the latest weapon in political warfare?

Whatever you may think of that particular theory the inescapable fact is that millions of ordinary God-fearing people in Britain became terrified of a disease that had killed just a handful of patients.

During 1986 and 1987 the mail I received from readers of my newspaper and magazine columns proved without any doubt that the propaganda campaign had adversely affected the lives of millions of men and women who had absolutely no risk at all of contracting the disease. So, for example, I received an extremely sad letter from a fifty-seven-year-old widow who had been to her doctor for an internal examination. She was worried that if the doctor had previously examined an Aids patient, she may have caught Aids. She told me that she wouldn't be going back to him again unless I could provide her with solid reassurance. Another letter came from a reader who wanted to know if her small son could have caught Aids from an insect bite. There were other letters from an old lady who wouldn't pat her dog in case she caught Aids from it, and a worried mother whose son wouldn't kiss her goodnight for fear of catching Aids. In May 1987 the National Association of Head Teachers warned that 'TV adverts warning against the dangers of Aids have frightened schoolchildren'.

And Michael Coles was by no means the only person to kill himself

– or commit murder – as a result of the Aids scaremongering. I haven't kept a comprehensive file of such cuttings but looking through my newspaper library I see that in April 1987 an eighteen-year-old boy called Lee Sands, living in Portsmouth, hanged himself after his family joked about him having Aids after a blood test to see if he had glandular fever. Since the total number of heterosexuals who have caught Aids in Britain and died is just six I strongly suspect that the scare campaign about Aids has killed more heterosexuals than the disease itself.

Whatever the reason may be for the distortion and the deceit the fact is that the publicity campaign has scared people unnecessarily and has attracted attention and resources away from areas where they are more desperately needed.

WHOOPING-COUGH VACCINE

The story of the whooping-cough vaccine provides us with another example of dishonesty and deceit in medicine.

There has been controversy about the whooping-cough vaccine for many years and the Department of Health and Social Security has consistently managed to convince the majority of medical staff to support the official line that the vaccine is both safe and effective. Once again the official DHSS line pays little attention to the facts. Put bluntly, the DHSS (on behalf of successive governments) has consistently lied about the risks and problems associated with the whooping-cough vaccine.

I'll explain exactly why I think that governments have lied (and this is not intended as a slight on any one political party – as far as I'm aware all political parties have followed exactly the same line on this matter) a little later. For the time being I'd like to concentrate solely on the facts.

The first point that should be made is that although official spokesmen claim otherwise, the whooping-cough vaccine has never had much of an influence on the number of children dying from whooping cough. The dramatic fall in the number of deaths caused by the disease came well before the vaccine was widely available and was, historians agree, the result of improved public health measures and, indirectly, the use of antibiotics.

It was in 1957 that the whooping-cough vaccine was first intro-duced nationally in Britain – although the vaccine was tried out in the late 1940s and early 1950s. But the incidence of whooping cough, and the number of children dying from the disease, had both fallen very considerably well before 1957. So, for example, while doctors reported 170,000 cases of whooping cough in 1950 they reported only about 80,000 cases in 1955. The introduction of the vaccine really didn't make very much, if any, difference to the fall in the incidence of the disease. Even today, thirty years after the introduction of the vaccine, whooping-cough cases are still running at about 1,000 a week in Britain.

Similarly, the figures show that the introduction of the vaccine had no effect on the number of children dying from whooping cough. The mortality rate associated with the disease had been falling appreciably since the early part of the twentieth century and rapidly since the 1930s and 1940s – showing a particularly steep decline after the introduction of the sulphonamide drugs. Whooping cough is undoubtedly an extremely unpleasant disease but it has not been a major killer for many years. The DHSS has frequently forecast fresh whooping-cough epidemics but none of the forecast epidemics has produced the devastation predicted.

My second point is that the whooping-cough vaccine is neither very efficient nor is it safe. The efficiency of the vaccine is of subsidiary interest – although thousands of children who have been vaccinated do still get the disease – the greatest controversy surrounds the safety of the vaccine. The DHSS has always claimed that serious adverse reactions to the whooping-cough vaccine are extremely rare and the official suggestion is that the risk of a child being brain damaged by the vaccine is no higher than one in 100,000. Now leaving aside the fact that I find a risk of one in 100,000 unacceptable, it is interesting to examine this figure a little more closely, for after a little research work it becomes clear that the figure of one in 100,000 is a guess.

Over the last decade or two, numerous researchers have studied the risks of brain damage following whooping-cough vaccination and their results make fascinating reading. Between 1960 and 1981, for example, nine reports were published showing that the risk of brain damage varied between one in 6,000 and one in 100,000. The average was a risk of one in 50,000. It is clear from these figures that the DHSS has simply chosen the figure which showed the whooping-cough vaccine to be least risky. Moreover, the one in 100,000 figure did not come from any rock solid research. It was itself an estimate – a guess.

These are just a couple of the important facts about the whooping-cough vaccine that have been ignored or overlooked or disguised by the DHSS. But they are not the only facts that have been distorted.

Although the DHSS consistently claims that whooping cough is a dangerous disease, the figures show that it is not the indiscriminate killer it is made out to be. Whooping cough causes around four

18

deaths a year in Britain. Compare that to approximately 300 deaths caused by tuberculosis and 100 deaths caused by meningitis. Most of the victims of whooping cough are babies under three months old. That fact is particularly important because the vaccine is never given to babies under three months old.

The truth about the whooping-cough vaccine is that it has always been a disaster. The vaccine has already been withdrawn in other countries because of the amount of brain damage associated with its use. In Japan, Sweden and West Germany the vaccine has been omitted from regular vaccination schedules. In America two out of three whooping-cough vaccine manufacturers have stopped making the vaccine because of the cost of lawsuits. On 6 December 1985 the *Journal of the American Medical Association* published a major report showing that the whooping-cough vaccine is, without doubt, linked to the development of serious brain damage. And even here in Britain the DHSS has been so worried about the vaccine that for ten years it has been paying research workers at Porton Down to search for ways to make a new, safer, more effective whooping-cough vaccine. At long last, after a £5 million research programme, a new vaccine is indeed being tested on children.

The final nail in the coffin lid is the fact that the British Government has already paid out compensation to the parents of some 800 children who have been brain damaged by the whooping-cough vaccine. Some parents who accepted damages a few years ago were given £10,000. More recently parents have been getting £20,000.

It is a startling fact that for many years now the whooping-cough vaccine has been killing or severely injuring more children than the disease itself. Since 1979 around 800 children (or their parents) have received money from the Government for vaccine-produced brain damage. In the same period less than 100 children have been killed by whooping cough. I think that makes the vaccine more dangerous than the disease. And that, surely, is quite unacceptable. So, why has the DHSS continued to encourage doctors to use the vaccine?

There are two possible explanations. The first explanation is the more generous of the two and concerns the Government's responsibility for the health of the community as a whole. The theory here is that by encouraging millions of parents to have their children vaccinated the Government can reduce the incidence of the disease in the community. In the long run this reduces the risk of there being any future epidemics of whooping cough. In other words the Government risks the lives of individual children for the good of the next generation.

The second, less charitable explanation is that the DHSS is looking after its own interests by continuing to claim that the whooping-cough vaccine is safe enough to use. In 1987 there were 258 sets of parents preparing to sue the DHSS for damages. They claim that the whooping-cough vaccine damaged their children. They are claiming something in the region of £250,000 each. If the DHSS withdrew the whooping-cough vaccine, it would be admitting that the vaccine was dangerous. And it would obviously lose its court cases. Such an admission would, therefore, cost it 258 times £250,000.

And that would be just the beginning for there are, you will remember, 800 sets of parents who have already received payments from the Government of either £10,000 or £20,000. If the DHSS admitted liability (and those payments did not include an admission of liability), then it is fair to assume that the DHSS would find itself with several hundred more lawsuits – and a damages bill running into billions of pounds.

Whatever explanation you consider most accurate the unavoidable fact is that the Government (in the form of the DHSS) has consistently lied about the whooping-cough vaccine, has distorted the truth and has deceived both the medical profession (for the majority of doctors and nurses who give these injections accept the recommendations made by the DHSS without question) and millions of parents.

The DHSS may have saved itself a tidy sum in damages. But the cost to the nation's health has been enormous. And this, remember, is merely one more example of the way in which the truth has been distorted by those whom we trust to provide us with honest, accurate advice about medicine and health care.

THE FOOD LOBBY

Few things are as important to our health as the food that we eat. Eat the wrong sort of foods and you increase your chances of developing one or both of the two biggest killers of the twentieth century – cancer and heart disease.

During the last couple of decades an enormous amount of money has been spent on research designed to find out which foodstuffs are responsible for which diseases. But as far as consumers are concerned there is still a good deal of confusion and controversy. Are animal fats bad for you? Does salt produce high blood pressure? How much fibre should the average daily diet contain? Listen to everything the so-called food experts say and you'll end up thoroughly confused because while one group will tell you one thing, another, equally eminent group, will say exactly the opposite.

In few areas of health are the lobbyists quite so effective. Imagine, for example, that a lone researcher in Sweden produces a piece of evidence showing that runner beans cause migraine. Because food and health are always of interest some newspaper or television correspondent will notice this research work and will print a paragraph or two detailing the results. At this point little harm will have been done. The research work will have affected relatively few people.

But by now the Runner Bean Marketing Board will have been alerted. Its advisers will scour the world's literature until they find an expert prepared to argue that runner beans are good for you. They may, if they are lucky, find a researcher in, say, Canada who believes that without runner beans daily we all run an increased risk of developing liver disease.

Frightened that the consumption of runner beans might be damaged by the original Swedish research, the Runner Bean Marketing Board (which is, of course, financed by the farmers whose livelihood depends upon the steady marketing and sale of runner beans) will pay for their foreign research scientist to go on an international tour. They'll arrange for him to hold press conferences and they'll reprint an expanded and well-illustrated copy of his research in a nicely bound booklet which they will post to doctors, dieticians, and reporters everywhere.

At this point the Broad Bean Marketing Board will start to get worried. They will see all this publicity for runner beans as a threat and they will look around for an expert or two of their very own. They'll probably come up with a specialist in Austria or Italy who believes that broad beans prevent heart disease or tooth decay or infertility. They will then provide him with an international platform from which to expound his views. And they won't be particularly worried if he also uses the massive publicity machine with which they have armed him to propound another dotty theory that carrots cause impotence and baldness. After all, their reasoning will be, if people stop buying carrots, they'll probably buy more broad beans.

The Carrot Marketing Board won't be too pleased by this new development, however, and they'll quickly launch a campaign of their own. In no time at all hundreds of experts from all around the world will be arguing with one another, producing quite different statistics, making all sorts of outrageous claims and ensuring that no one listens to anything that the doctors say. The whole business of mass communications becomes devalued.

The food industry was, I suspect, one of the first big international industries to realize that you can buy any number of apparently reputable medical experts with a few grants and a fistful of airline

21

tickets to conferences in the Bahamas. And few industries do more harm with their lobbying. Between them these very professional lobbyists must have been responsible for thousands of avoidable deaths.

To give a more specific example take the case of animal fat. The way in which our awareness of the importance (and danger) of animal fat has been confused highlights the awesome power, enviable effectiveness, and disastrous consequences of this type of enthusiastic, no-holds-barred commercial lobbying. This isn't just a case of large companies fighting for a larger slice of the commercial cake. It is big business ruthlessly distorting the truth and callously exposing millions to a dangerous and potentially lethal lifestyle.

Look at the independent scientific evidence about animal fat and there is no doubt that animal fat is the one foodstuff of which most of us eat too much. In an editorial in *Update* in June 1987 Dr Geoffrey Rose, Professor of Epidemiology at the London School of Hygiene and Tropical Medicine, pointed out that 'the amount of fats – especially saturated fats – consumed by the average British person is highly dangerous. The World Health Organization, the British Cardiac Society, the Royal College of Physicians, the British Heart Foundation, the British Nutrition Foundation, and the DHSS all agree that our present national diet is an unhealthy one'. Back in 1953 it was shown that there was a convincing correlation between a high intake of animal fat and the development of heart disease. Over twenty independent, major scientific and medical committees around the world have agreed that we should eat less fatty meat, less butter, less cream, and fewer eggs. I don't know of any independent expert group or committee which disagrees with that conclusion. In 1982 even the World Health Organization, a bureaucratic beast which lumbers slowly towards conclusions, published a recommendation of its own advising people to cut down on fat. And in many countries around the world a reduction in the consumption of animal fat has led to a noticeable reduction in the incidence of heart disease.

But in Britain confusion and chaos have remained. The consumption of animal fat has remained high. And the incidence of heart disease has not fallen. Indeed, Britain, where animal fat consumption is high, has now got one of the worst heart-attack rates in the world. Every year thousands of young men and women in their thirties and forties die prematurely because they have been encouraged to eat unlimited quantities of fat. The credit for this mass annual slaughter must go to the farmers and food manufacturers who have between them organized a powerful and effective lobby to disguise and distort the truth about animal fats.

Since they have an obvious commercial interest in ensuring that we all continue to eat lots of butter, lots of eggs, and lots of fatty meat, and to wash it all down with lots of full-cream milk British farmers and food manufacturers have joined together to pay for a number of extremely effective and cruelly ruthless propaganda organizations. These organizations do their work in a number of ways.

They bombard doctors with a seemingly endless series of booklets and leaflets written and prepared by their own hired experts. The Butter Information Council has in recent years, for example, hired such eminent and well-known science writers as Dr Clive Wood and Dr Malcolm Carruthers to prepare material for them. Journalists are also bombarded with this material and with the names of experts who can be quoted or interviewed.

In addition, of course, these lobbying and public-relations groups also buy huge amounts of advertising space to put forward their views. In 1985, for example, the National Dairy Council – promoting milk – spent more on advertising than any food company. Their account for the year came to £8,765,400. The Butter Information Council spent just under £3,000,000.

Spending money like this on advertising gives the food lobby groups a chance to use their wealth and spending power to try and suppress the views of those who would argue a different, more independent line. So, for example, after I appeared on TV AM and gave my opinion that a high fat diet containing too much butter and milk could lead to heart disease, the Head of Features at the television station received a letter from a Mr Christopher Bird, Chief Executive of the Butter Information Council.

After commenting on my remarks about butter, Mr Bird wrote, 'On the day that this was transmitted the Butter Information Council was about to commit £54,372 to a burst of advertising on TV AM. I think that you can probably well imagine that this decision came under review in the light of such remarks.' Fortunately, in that instance the lawyer for TV AM wrote back to point out to Mr Bird that 'the placement of advertising spots is quite separate to the editorial content of the programme items'.

After that particular programme the Director of Programmes at TV AM also received a letter about my contribution. His letter came from a Dr Alexander L. Macnair who has an address in Wimpole Street and who described himself in his letter as an independent consultant. Dr Macnair, who disagreed with my conclusions about butter, did not mention that his work has included advising both the Butter Information Council and the Eggs Authority. Neither did Dr Macnair mention these commercial links when, a few months later, he wrote to *The Times* about diet and heart disease.

23

Over the last few years I have received or been the subject of countless letters and telephone calls from the Butter Information Council, the Eggs Authority, the Milk Marketing Board, and other similar powerful pressure groups.

It is my experience that any newspaper, magazine or television company that includes material suggesting that there is a link between fat consumption and heart disease will be bombarded with material proposing an opposite point of view. There is nothing at all wrong with this, of course, when the letters and phone calls are clearly seen to come from a pressure group. But it is frightening that the large commercial pressure groups should be able to find apparently 'independent' consultants to write on their behalf. And it is also frightening to realize that these pressure groups are not averse to using what seems to me to be lightly veiled commercial blackmail in their attempts to suppress what the majority of truly independent experts see as the truth.

THE TOBACCO INDUSTRY

In 1984 the Chief Medical Officer at the DHSS reported that smoking is 'by far the largest avoidable health hazard in Britain today and causes about 100,000 deaths in the UK each year'. A previous Chief Medical Officer at the DHSS once described the cigarette as 'the most lethal instrument devised by man for peaceful use'.

According to official statistics, the majority of the thousands of people who have major surgery in Britain are smokers. Ninety-five per cent of all patients with serious arterial disease of the legs are smokers and twenty per cent of the 180,000 people who die of coronary artery disease every year do so because they smoke.

The list of diseases associated with tobacco smoking seems to grow annually. There are the respiratory disorders such as asthma and bronchitis. Chest infections are particularly common among smokers. Sinus troubles such as sinusitis and catarrh are caused or made worse by tobacco as are many gum and tooth disorders. Of the problems which affect the stomach, indigestion, gastritis and peptic ulcers have all been identified as being exacerbated by smoking. Many circulatory problems, raised blood pressure, arterial blockages, and strokes are all known to be tobacco-related. Dr Michael Russell of the Addiction Research Unit at the Institute of Psychiatry in London has even pointed out that exhaled cigarette smoke could kill as many as 1,000 non-smokers every year.

Despite all this well-documented evidence, countless millions still smoke regularly. And the British tobacco industry still spends £100 million a year on advertising and sponsorship. Although the British Government banned cigarette advertising on television in 1965, the industry's promotional activities have proved remarkably successful. While they are banned from advertising directly on British television, a number of tobacco companies ensure plenty of exposure for their brand names on television by sponsoring sporting events.

In 1986–7 the tobacco and alcohol industries sponsored events in the following sports: American football, angling, athletics, badminton, basketball, bowls, boxing, canoeing, cricket, croquet, curling, cycling, darts, golf, greyhound racing, handball, hockey, horse jumping, horse racing, ice hockey, ice skating, motorcycling, motor racing, motor rallying, pool, rowing, rugby league, rugby union, skiing, snooker, soccer, street hockey, surfing, tennis, windsurfing, and yachting. And I have no doubt that this advertising is effective. In a report published in the *Health Education Journal* in 1984 Frank Ledwith, research fellow in the Department of Education at the University of Manchester, reported on a survey which involved 880 secondary-school children in the city.

Ledwith found that children are most aware of the cigarette brands which are most frequently associated with sponsored sporting events on TV. He concluded that 'children's TV viewing of a recent snooker championship sponsored by one cigarette manufacturer was positively correlated with the proportion of children associating that brand, and other brands used in TV sponsorship, with sport'. After conducting a second survey following a snooker championship sponsored by another cigarette manufacturer Ledwith reported that 'TV sports sponsorship by tobacco manufacturers acts as cigarette advertising to children and therefore circumvents the law banning cigarette advertisements on TV'.

Not surprisingly, the tobacco industry argues that publicity doesn't attract new smokers, but merely persuades smokers to change brands. The Advertising Association (which cynics might assume has a vested interest in defending the interests of the tobacco industry) claims that advertising expenditure has not had any significant influence on the total size of the cigarette market over the last twenty years, and claims that 'advertising does not stimulate or maintain cigarette consumption levels'.

The World Health Organization's Expert Committee on Smoking Control Strategies in Developing Countries finds this argument unconvincing. In 1982 it reported that 'some pro-smoking advertisements do not even mention a brand name' and that 'tobacco companies enjoying a complete monopoly in a country none the less advertise.' But whatever the World Health Organization may say, and whatever anti-smoking groups may say, the pro-smoking lobby marches on. It is a powerful force in Britain.

In other countries braver and more forceful stances have been taken against smoking. A study of smoking in fifteen countries, published in the British Government's own official journal *Health Trends*, recently concluded that 'the countries which have evolved the most stringent anti-smoking policies (such as Norway and Finland) are among the lowest consumers of tobacco'. But the British Government has been reluctant to take further action to control smoking. In the budget in 1987 the Chancellor did not even increase the amount of tax on cigarettes – a well-proven method of encouraging people to cut down their smoking.

It is difficult to avoid the conclusion that the Government is unwilling to annoy or hamper an industry which provides the Exchequer with £4,000 million a year in taxes. Indeed, the Government is so keen to support and encourage the tobacco industry that it helps to subsidize the growing of tobacco. The European Economic Community's Agricultural Policy gives European tobacco farmers a $667 million a year subsidy. And that means that every tax-paying non-smoker in Europe is helping to support the world's richest and most successful industry of addiction.

True cynics also argue that the Government does not try too hard to control the tobacco industry not simply because of the £4,000 million a year revenue it receives, but also because without the high annual death toll associated with tobacco the size of Britain's elderly population would be even greater.

THE ALCOHOL INDUSTRY

According to Hyman and Beaumont in an article entitled 'Identifying the Problem Drinker', published in *Occupational Safety and Health* in 1984, about four per cent of the population in England and Wales and ten per cent of the population in Scotland are problem drinkers – their drinking harms their health, occupation, social life or domestic life.

In February 1987 Dr E. G. Lucas, Consultant Psychiatrist at King's College Hospital in London and Adviser in Mental Health to the Health and Safety Executive, contributed an editorial to the *British Medical Journal* in which he pointed out that alcohol-related sickness and absenteeism may cost industry £641 million a year while accidents and poor performance related to alcohol may cost an impressive £1.5 billion.

In 1979 the Thirty-second World Health Assembly declared that 'problems related to alcohol, and particularly to its excessive consumption, rank among the world's major public health problems' and 'constitute serious hazards for human health, welfare and life'.

In my book *Addicts and Addictions* (published in 1986) I pointed out that alcohol causes between a third and a half of all road deaths in developed countries. It also causes about a third of all accidents at work. It adversely affects the abilities of politicians and businessmen, of doctors and entertainers. It is involved in a third of all divorces and a third of all child-abuse cases.

In America it has been confirmed that more than seventy-five per cent of police time is spent on alcohol-related crimes, that the vast majority of criminals are heavy drinkers and that about one-half of all murders are alcohol related, in that either the victim or the murderer had been drinking. In Britain research reported in the *British Journal of Addiction* in 1983 showed that sixty-four per cent of all people arrested had been drinking in the four hours prior to their arrest, while among people arrested between 10 p.m. and 2 a.m. ninety-three per cent had been drinking heavily. Even among the under eighteen-year-olds arrested sixty-five per cent had been drinking. Alcohol is a significant factor in about 1,000 arrests every day in Britain. And the problem is getting worse. In Britain the consumption of alcohol has doubled in the last thirty years.

The major risk for a drinker is, of course, that he will become an alcoholic – a drinker trapped by his need to keep drinking. According to the World Health Organization between one and ten per cent of the world's population can be properly described as alcoholics. Experts argue about just how much a drinker needs to consume to become an alcoholic, but the consensus of opinion seems to be that if you drink five pints of beer or a third of a pint of whisky a day then you are in trouble. Something like one in every three drinkers is already in this category or is heading for it. Once someone has become an alcoholic then he will be four times as likely to die in any given year as a non-drinker of the same age, sex and economic status.

Many people still believe that the only organ likely to be damaged by drinking is the liver. But that just isn't true. People who drink too much risk developing cancer, stomach ulcers and muscle wastage – as well as liver disease. Women who drink too much and who get pregnant run a real risk of having low birth weight or backward babies. They also run an increased risk of developing physical problems, such as liver disease, for the female body is physiologically more vulnerable than the male body to the adverse effects of alcohol.

It is, however, the effects that alcohol has on the brain that make it particularly dangerous. Alcohol is detectable in the brain within half a minute of a glass being emptied. Once alcohol gets to the brain the

27

first effect it has is that of a depressant. If you drink a small amount, the depressant effect seems to work most noticeably on the part of the brain that controls your tendency to get excited. With the controls depressed you become more excitable and talkative. That's why we consider alcohol to be a social lubricant. Social and personal inhibitions are lifted by alcohol and most people, when they have had a drink or two, become much looser and less restricted by social convention.

However, at the same time as alcohol is depressing inhibitions it also has other effects. The brain's ability to concentrate on information, understand messages that it is receiving, and make judgements on those messages will diminish. Reflexes will go and although the individual won't be aware of it his ability to link sensory input to muscular function will be badly distorted. The person who has been drinking will think that he will be able to talk, dance or drive a car more efficiently than normal whereas in fact his ability to do these things will be adversely affected. Eventually the depressant effect of alcohol affects other areas of brain function. In the end the individual who has drunk too much will appear drunken and will probably fall into a deep sleep.

The results of all this damage are difficult to overestimate. In France, where the consumption of alcohol per head is the highest in the world, ten per cent of all deaths are directly due to the excessive consumption of alcohol. In Britain twenty per cent of male admissions to general medical wards are related to the use of alcohol. In 1980, for example, approximately 500,000 admissions to general medical wards were caused by excessive drinking. These figures sound so startling as to be impossible but numerous independent researchers have shown them to be accurate. For example, in the *Journal of the Royal Society of Medicine* in March 1986 a team of six doctors from St Charles' Hospital in London published an article entitled 'Detecting Alcohol Consumption as a Cause of Emergency General Medical Admissions'. They showed that in their general medical unit twenty-seven per cent of admissions were attributed to alcohol consumption while seventeen per cent of their beds were occupied by patients suffering from problems caused by alcohol consumption. Alcohol is, without a doubt, one of the most destructive forces in Britain today. A joint report by the British Medical Association and Action on Alcohol Abuse reported that in addition to the illness and disability caused by alcohol the number of deaths directly attributable to alcohol abuse is now around 6,500 per year. To put this into perspective it is perhaps worth pointing out that official DHSS figures show that the number of deaths related to heroin and morphine abuse in Britain is around fifty a year.

It isn't difficult to find a reason for our growing alcohol problem. The alcohol industry in Britain is large, rich and extremely powerful. The production, marketing and selling of alcohol employs over 750,000 people. Alcohol exports earn the country over £1,000 million a year and the tax raised on alcohol exceeds £5,000 million a year. The alcohol industry spends over £100 million a year persuading us to buy its products. There are remarkably few restrictions on advertising and the industry's copywriters have succeeded in making alcohol one of the standard Christmas gifts. Not that all the money spent on promotion goes on direct advertising – the alcohol industry also employs lobbyists whose job it is to persuade our politicians to keep taxes down. The industry has been remarkably effective at this – in the 1987 budget the tax on alcohol was not increased at all. (Nor, as I've already pointed out, was the tax on tobacco increased).

Like the tobacco industry the alcohol industry spends a considerable amount of money on sports sponsorship and has found this type of advertising to be extremely effective. So far, well over sixty different sports have accepted sponsorship money from one or both of these industries. Badminton, bowls, canoeing, croquet, handball, hockey, cricket, horse racing, ice hockey, ice skating, motor racing, rugby league, rugby union, snooker, soccer, and tennis are all among the sports scrabbling for blood money.

All this advertising and sponsorship is so effective that according to an article entitled 'Alcohol Use in Britain: How Much Is Too Much?' written by W. M. Saunders, Senior Lecturer and Director of the Alcohol Studies Centre in Paisley, Scotland, and published in the *Health Education Journal* in 1984, in any one week over seventy-five per cent of men and fifty per cent of women will consume alcohol. In 1982 the people of Britain drank some 1,350 million gallons of beer, 35 million proof gallons of spirits and 106 million gallons of wine. Every single day we spend tens of millions of pounds on alcohol. As a nation we spend more money on alcohol than we spend on clothing or the running of our motor cars. An incredible 7.4 per cent of all consumer expenditure goes on alcohol.

The fact that alcohol can be obtained legally and easily means that millions who would never dream of using an illegal prop are happy to use it as an aid in dealing with stress or pressure. Alcohol is, indeed, the one drug that is regularly sanitized by the political and ecclesiastical establishments. Catholics, Jews and Protestants all celebrate religious festivals with alcohol. Socially, just about every dinner or toast, speech or function is celebrated with alcohol. We even launch a new boat by smashing a bottle of champagne over its bow. This social acceptability means that alcohol is usually the first substance most law-abiding citizens reach for when things start getting tough.

It isn't only better and more effective advertising that has helped to increase the amount of alcohol that is consumed. In recent years alcohol has become ever more widely available. These days it is sold freely in self-service stores and supermarkets. You can pick it up and take it home with the washing powder and the cat food. No one will notice or think anything of it. In my view making alcohol freely available in shops has been a major factor in the rapid rise in the number of female alcoholics in our society. Ten years ago there were eight men to every one woman with a real drinking problem. Today, there are only three times as many men with a drinking problem. Anyone working in a clinic for alcoholics or any member of Alcoholics Anonymous will confirm that alcoholism has become rife among women aged between thirty and fifty. On any nice, neat modern housing estate, where there are countless women locked into loneliness and embittered by boredom, there will be hundreds of alcoholics hiding behind neatly painted doors. They start drinking through boredom, anxiety, frustration and loneliness. To begin with it is easy. There is no difficulty in getting supplies and there may even be some social cachet in being able to drink men under the table. By the time the addiction has taken hold the woman drinker will be consumed with guilt and shame. Once those destructive and inescapable emotions are added to her original loneliness, boredom and frustration her drinking problem will be complete. She will be a prisoner of her habit, locked into continuing despair.

The bizarre thing is that despite the size of our current alcohol abuse problem virtually nothing is done to help stop the problem growing or to help treat the hundreds of thousands who desperately need guidance. Indeed, many who might be expected to do something positive to help do nothing – or even deny that a problem exists. In a publication entitled *The Impact of Advertising on the United Kingdom Alcoholic Drink Market*, published in 1983 by the Advertising Association, Dr L. W. Hagan and M. J. Waterson claim that 'only a very small fraction of the population can be classed as alcoholics or as abusing alcohol in a serious manner.'

Rather than doing anything to control the sale and use of alcohol the British Government seems determined to encourage the alcohol industry. Those who successfully sell alcohol are given huge salaries, expensive perks, index-linked pensions and awards in the honours list. A report by Action on Alcohol Abuse, published in 1986, produced some figures which show just how interested the Government is in fighting our tobacco and alcohol problems. The report showed that for each tobacco-related premature death the Government spends £35. For each death related to the abuse of alcohol the

Government spends £344 on trying to help patients and stop people drinking too much. But for each death caused by illegal drugs the Government spends £1,700,000 on propaganda outlining the hazards of illegal drug use. It is difficult to avoid the conclusion that the Government is only prepared to take action to control drug abuse when there is not likely to be a price to pay in terms of lost revenues.

Those who work for and represent these industries present the truly unacceptable face of capitalism and we should reserve our contempt for them and their efforts. But we should, perhaps, reserve our greatest contempt for our politicians who steadfastly refuse to do anything to help cut down the amount of death and disability produced by alcohol and tobacco abuse. Between them the industrialists and the politicians have killed more Britons than Hitler and his generals.

THE DRUGS INDUSTRY

In my first book, *The Medicine Men*, published in 1975 I described my concern at the way the drugs industry promotes its products and uses modern marketing skills – together with old-fashioned bribery and corruption – to persuade doctors to prescribe the latest and most expensive products.

Since then nothing much has changed. If anything, things have got worse and today the drugs industry has a very tight hold over the medical profession. Most practising doctors get most or all of their postgraduate education from sources sponsored or paid for directly by the drugs industry. The British Medical Association receives hundreds of thousands of pounds every year from the drugs industry. And thousands of individual doctors allow themselves to be 'bought' by companies aggressively pushing new products.

The drugs industry has even reached into the heart of the medical establishment – the General Medical Council – and members of the Council (which regulates disciplinary procedures within the medical profession) have admitted that they receive large sums of money from drug companies. Doctors in powerful positions on the GMC have received money for research and for expensive overseas trips.

It is, perhaps, hardly surprising that as one of the drug industry's most vocal and persistent critics I have on numerous occasions been 'reported' to the disciplinary committee of the GMC or threatened with disciplinary action. So far the GMC hasn't managed to find a good excuse for disciplining me. But I suspect that they'll keep trying.

Not that the British Medical Association and the General Medical

Council are the only parts of the medical establishment to have become badly contaminated by links with the drugs industry. It is probably impossible to find any part of the medical establishment that hasn't accepted considerable amounts of drug-industry money or that hasn't allowed itself to become directly associated with the industry.

Take, for example, the Royal College of General Practitioners. As its name suggests the RCGP represents the specific academic and professional interests of Britain's general practitioners. The RCGP hasn't been around for long but that hasn't stopped it developing a close working relationship with what most independent financial experts consider to be one of the world's most efficient, ruthless, powerful and profitable industries. So, for example, the Royal College has created an organization called the Medicine Surveillance Organization which exists to help organize and run drugs surveillance projects for drug companies.

In 1984 outside observers and some members of the College complained about the MSO being hired by Hoffmann–La Roche to research a new benzodiazepine tranquillizer and being hired by another company to investigate a new and relatively untried pain-killer. The RCGP's business offshoot offered to pay doctors who helped a fee of between £60 and £70 as a 'contribution towards expenses and a token recognition of their contribution to the college's research programme'.

Dr Joe Collier, Deputy Editor of the *Drugs and Therapeutics Bulletin* (one of the very few drugs journals in existence which doesn't accept any drug-industry advertising) dismissed the trials as 'unlikely to produce any clinically helpful results'.

Those doctors who were responsible for forging these close links between the RCGP and the drugs industry should, perhaps, have been aware that drug-industry sponsored research is often done more to promote the drug and to encourage doctors to start prescribing the product than to obtain truly useful results. Dr Bill Inman, one of Britain's most experienced drug observers, runs the highly respected and independent Prescription Event Monitoring Scheme. He has had harsh things to say about research done by drug companies on newly marketed products, and has described this sort of work as nothing more than a ploy to buy a market for a drug. One of the directors of the Medicine Surveillance Organization (the RCGP's subsidiary) was Dr Clifford Kay. According to a report in *Medical News* in November 1984 Dr Kay admitted that a number of mistakes had been made in the protocol of one of the trials planned by the organization for a new non-steroidal anti-inflammatory drug. The trial was criticized in the *Drug and Therapeutics Bulletin* which pointed out that 'participating doctors will provide or prescribe the drug to patients to whom they might otherwise have given an established mild analgesic for conditions which improve steadily without treatment.' And it alleged that 'the significance of the frequency of adverse effects will be impossible to interpret'. Dr Kay admitted that MSO was probably wrong in offering to pay GPs £6 per patient to provide reports.

Of course, not all drug company promotional money is spent on marketing trials of spurious value (see also p. 34). Much of their money is spent on straightforward advertising and on wining and dining doctors in an attempt to buy their loyalty. Every year the drugs industry in Britain spends around £200 million on selling its drugs to doctors. That means that each year drug companies spend around £5,000 persuading each family doctor to prescribe their products. They give him free gifts, they send him free magazines, they take him out to lunch (I know of GPs who haven't paid for a meal in a restaurant in years), they bombard him with leaflets, and they pay for him to go abroad to 'conferences' (which are, oddly enough, always held in exotic places like Miami or Hong Kong. They rarely hold conferences in Manchester or Reading). Most of the drug company representatives who promote drugs to doctors (and who are, therefore, directly responsible for 'educating' doctors in Britain) have no official medical training at all. They are merely indoctrinated with basic information about a small number of drugs and then encouraged to pass that information on to the doctors they meet.

In contrast, the NHS spends about £70 per doctor per year on providing information about new drugs and on teaching doctors about the problems and side effects associated with modern treatments. And the average doctor probably spends about £5 a year on his own education. One new textbook every five years is probably an over-optimistic estimate of the average GP's commitment to self-improvement. It is an alarming thought that most of the doctors in practice today qualified before the contraceptive pill was generally available and completed their training in pre-Valium times. Most of the drugs GPs prescribe have been introduced since they qualified and information about new ones arrives through the letter box every day. Most doctors are twenty-four when they qualify so a doctor now aged forty probably qualified in 1970. A doctor who is now fifty will have qualified before oral contraception, heart, liver, kidney or lung transplantation, and tranquillizing drugs were introduced. He will have qualified before at least eighty per cent of the drugs he prescribes were introduced. And he will have qualified before drug side effects and hazards were widely recognized.

It is hardly surprising that the majority of doctors in practice today

33

are badly informed and uncritical. As I wrote in 1975 in *The Medicine Men*, it is difficult to see how a profession that takes its instructions from a trade can continue to call itself a profession. Or to put it another way, if lawyers allowed burglars to make our laws, then I suspect that our respect for the legal profession would reach a new low.

Not that the drug companies always get away with things these days. In the last year or two there have been a number of attempts to curb their traditionally excessive enthusiasm for their new products. The trouble is, however, that these attempts at discipline merely highlight the arrogance of those in the industry. So, for example, in the last week or two of 1986 there were three quite separate instances which illustrated the ways in which the drug companies now work.

First, Roussel Laboratories and its medical director Dr Christopher Good were convicted by a jury of issuing misleading advertisements about an anti-arthritis drug called Surgam. The advertisements appeared in the *British Medical Journal*. Roussel was fined £20,000 and Good was fined £1,000 although both lodged appeals.

Second, the drug company Bayer UK was suspended from the Association of the British Pharmaceutical Industry for allegedly bringing discredit on the whole pharmaceutical industry. The offence? People working for Bayer had been reported to have given doctors money and gifts to conduct bogus drug trials. Doctors participating in the bogus trials were said to have received payments towards colour television sets and trips to medical conferences in the United States of America.

It is, perhaps, interesting to note that none of the doctors alleged to have taken part in these bogus trials was threatened with disciplinary action. And, of course, the drugs produced by Roussel and Bayer were both allowed to remain on the market.

The third scandal of that month linked to the drugs industry concerned Dr Ian Robertson, an honorary consultant at Glasgow's Western Infirmary Blood Pressure Unit. Dr Robertson, who worked for the Medical Research Council, resigned after it was revealed that while working for the MRC he had received money from at least half a dozen leading drug companies.

These were by no means isolated cases. Hardly a week goes by without fresh scandals about the drug industry being brought to light. For example, in March 1987 the Code of Practice Committee of the Association of the British Pharmaceutical Industry found Pfizer Ltd guilty of making misleading claims about a product used in the treatment of high blood pressure. The Committee also found International Laboratories Ltd in breach of the code for making exaggerated claims about one of its products and similarly Gist-Brocades

34

Pharmaceuticals for producing an unbalanced report of a medical society meeting without permission and also including it in an advertisement for a product called De-Nol. Another company, Organon Laboratories Ltd, was also found in breach of the code for advertising an antidepressant drug directly to the public.

It is interesting to note that another drug company was found not guilty for organizing a competition in which 1,000 clocks were given away as prizes. The Committee decided that the prizes (only available to doctors) were of some relevance to the practice of medicine since doctors need to know the time.

These frequent lapses by drug companies are bad enough, but they merely illustrate the tip of a very extensive iceberg. It is the subtler techniques and tricks which we should, perhaps, be more worried about. For example, the CIBA Foundation (a registered charity) runs a register of spokesmen for newspaper and television writers who want advice on any medical or scientific topics. Am I, I wonder, being unreasonably paranoid in suspecting that a journalist who calls the service will be given the name and telephone number of a doctor whose views are not offensive to CIBA?

According to a letter published in the *British Medical Journal* in December 1986 another drug company offers to write doctors' scientific papers for them. The doctor has only to send in raw data and tell the company what journal he would like the paper to appear in. The company will then prepare the paper, provide the references and print copies. The company decides which data to highlight and which to omit. A company employee will also write the introduction to the paper and draw the conclusions.

If an independent scientific journal cannot be persuaded to print the paper, I have no doubt that, if the paper were suitably useful, the company would be able to put the original author in touch with a journal that would print the paper and charge the company a fee. There is nothing new in this. When I first described this practice in my book *Paper Doctors* in 1977 *The Journal of International Medical Research* was charging companies £85 per printed page for scientific papers.

These are, of course, all fairly minor examples of the way that the drugs industry works. It is, however, also important to realize that there is a wider implication. The drug companies do not merely use questionable marketing techniques to help them promote individual products; they also use their power and their money to help ensure that medical treatment remains drug-based.

In the last decade or two an enormous amount of evidence has been produced to show that the majority of medical problems can be treated best without drugs. For example, although it was once believed that high blood pressure always needed drug treatment, it is now widely acknowledged that the majority of patients who have high blood pressure do not need to take pills for the rest of their lives. Their hypertension can be controlled if they lose weight, cut down their salt intake, stop smoking, and learn how to relax properly.

Despite the availability of this evidence, however, most doctors still persist in treating high blood pressure with pills. And the Medical Research Council's long-running research into high blood pressure has concentrated on drug therapies rather than safer, cheaper, and more effective alternatives. (This, incidentally, helps to explain why I and some other observers found the Robertson scandal so sinister.)

The power of the drugs industry also helps to explain why so many doctors still persist in treating pain with pills rather than with TENS machines. The story of just how the drugs industry has managed to suppress the TENS machine makes chilling reading.

TENS machines are pocket-sized, battery-operated stimulators which send out a continuous series of electrical pulses. The name stands for Transcutaneous Electrical Nerve Stimulation. Have you ever noticed how rubbing a sore spot can relieve pain? Rubbing works by increasing the number of non-painful messages travelling towards the spinal cord. This mass of messages blocks the route to the brain and prevents pain messages getting through. Bang your elbow and you'll unconsciously start rubbing it because you know that it will help. The TENS machines work along the same lines.

During the last ten years an impressive number of projects have been undertaken and have shown without doubt that TENS machines are cheap, safe, portable and effective ways of controlling pain.

In a study conducted with patients suffering from rheumatoid arthritis it was found that TENS equipment produced pain relief in up to ninety-five per cent of patients. In other experiments it was found that TENS even managed to produce relief in patients who had received no relief from any other pain-relieving technique or drug. Pain experts have shown that TENS machines provide relief for sixty-five to eighty per cent of all pain patients in the short term and long term relief for between thirty per cent and fifty per cent of patients.

For example, according to Professor John Thompson, Professor of Pharmacology at the University of Newcastle-upon-Tyne, who is consultant clinical pharmacologist for the Newcastle Health Authority and consultant in charge at the pain relief clinic at the Royal Victoria Infirmary in Newcastle, short-term improvement after using a TENS machine may be between eighty and ninety per cent with a very respectable thirty-five per cent of patients still benefiting from pain relief after two years' use.

It has been shown that the TENS machine, which is cheap to buy and run and which produces extremely few side effects (none of them particularly dangerous) is good for relieving many types of pain. A report from doctors working in Glasgow, published in the *Annals of Rheumatic Disease* in 1984 showed that they are extremely good for the treatment of the pain produced by osteoarthritic knees. A report from Montreal, mentioned in *Rheumatology in Practice* in 1984 showed that they are good in the treatment of soft-tissue rheumatism. A Cambridge group reported that TENS helps patients suffering from painful shoulders. In fact they have been shown to work for phantom limb pain, arthritis of all kinds, cancer pain, as well as the pain that sometimes develops after shingles. A large study done in Sweden showed that TENS is the only painkiller required by seventy-five per cent of women in labour. Other work has shown that TENS works well for patients recovering from surgery, too. (I described TENS machines in more detail in my book *Natural Pain Control* in 1986.)

But despite this mass of evidence showing that TENS machines work and are safe, very few patients have ever heard of them and very few doctors use them. There is, of course, a simple explanation for this apparent paradox. Drug companies don't like the idea of small, portable, cheap machines being available which can be used to treat pain without side effects or danger. The drug companies know that if there were a TENS machine in every medicine cabinet the sales of pain relievers (one of industry's major sources of revenue) would collapse overnight. If TENS machines became widely available, the cost to the industry would probably run into billions of pounds.

So, how has the drugs industry managed to suppress a simple and effective piece of equipment? Why have few doctors and even fewer patients ever heard of a TENS machine – let alone actually seen one? There are two explanations.

First, the drugs industry now has such a powerful hold over the training of doctors that there is no risk of them stumbling across TENS machines at a postgraduate lecture or a conference on pain relief. I spent ten years working as a general practitioner and I don't think I was ever invited to a lecture or meeting that wasn't sponsored by a drug company. TENS machines, like other non-drug remedies such as mental relaxation, are not discussed at sponsored meetings.

The second explanation is less subtle. The drugs industry has done its best deliberately to suppress the news about TENS machines and has successfully managed to prevent the production of TENS machines ever really taking off. If you think I'm being cynical, then consider this short, true story.

37

In 1970 two men, Norman Hagfors and Stanley McDonald, working in the basement of Mr Hagfor's home in Minneapolis, invented one of the earliest types of TENS machines. With the aid of electrical components bought at a local hardware store Hagfors and McDonald built a small device which blocked pain simply through electrodes stuck on to the patient's skin. Within three years the company the two men had formed, Stimulation Technology Inc., was selling almost a million dollars' worth of the devices annually.

Then, in 1974, one of the world's biggest drug companies bought out the company for $1.3 million, promising the two inventors a share of future profits. But, according to Hagfors and McDonald, the drug company did little or nothing to promote the product to pain sufferers, even though clinical trials had been successful. You may, or may not, be surprised to hear that the company in question makes a tremendous amount of money from the sale of painkilling tablets.

THE BRITISH MEDICAL ASSOCIATION – THE PATIENT'S ENEMY

These days medical journalists don't seem able to write medical stories without first obtaining a statement from the British Medical Association. If there is a story about teenage girls being given the contraceptive pill, the reporters will loyally quote the BMA's 'official' view. If there is a story about the NHS then the ubiquitous BMA spokesmen will be there telling us what the BMA thinks of it all. The BMA is never short of an opinion and every opinion is an 'official' one.

There is, I believe, a great danger in all this, for the British Medical Association is the doctors' trade union. It is not an independent body and its spokesmen cannot be relied upon to give an objective opinion on any medical problem. The BMA exists to protect the interests of its members; to fight for better pay and conditions for doctors. Talking to a BMA spokesman about health matters is like talking to a National Union of Mineworkers' spokesman on energy matters. The answer is bound to be biased and designed to support a particular point of view, as well as to protect a specific group of people. BMA spokesmen tend to be pompous and to sound authoritative, but in fact they have no official status whatsoever.

I think it is important to make this clear because the BMA has managed to carve for itself a position of great authority and responsibility. Its spokesmen (there are hundreds of people who describe themselves as BMA spokesmen and women, some are elected, some paid; the majority speak without any reference to the membership of the union) are prone to making sweeping and definitive statements which are then regarded by politicians and public alike as 'law'. And the sad and tragic truth is that by and large the BMA's interests and the public's interests rarely coincide. Indeed, I would argue that the BMA is probably the worst enemy that patients have.

The inescapable basic truth is that every time a BMA spokesman makes a statement his words will be influenced not by what is right for the country, the NHS or the ordinary patient, but by what is going to be good for doctors. Let me illustrate my argument with some specific examples.

First, there is the fact that the BMA has consistently opposed the provision of an easier complaints system for patients. Anyone who has ever tried to make a complaint about a doctor will know just how incomprehensible and impenetrable the present system is.

Recognizing the problem the British Government recently decided that it would make it easier for patients to complain about their doctors. The Government's plan was overwhelmingly rejected by the BMA. A simpler complaints system might be fairer and better for patients, but it certainly wouldn't be better for doctors.

Secondly, there is the fact that the BMA doesn't approve of patients having open access to their medical records. For some time now many politicians and patients' groups have argued that patients should be allowed complete freedom to see their medical records. Some doctors even agree with my rather radical suggestion that everyone would benefit if patients were allowed to keep their medical records at home. But the BMA has long opposed access to medical records. The 'official' line was that it would be bad for patients to be able to read their own notes – they might discover something alarming, they might misunderstand medical jargon or they might take offence at personal remarks. Bad for patients? Or bad for doctors? In the summer of 1987 the British Medical Association did agree in principle to back a code of practice giving patients the right to see their medical records. According to a report in *The Independent* the BMA made this decision after receiving a letter from Dr Ronald Oliver, the Deputy Chief Medical Officer at the Department of Health which gave a between-the-lines warning that the Government could not forever resist public demands for access to medical records.

Thirdly, the BMA has made it clear that it doesn't want information about doctors to be freely available to patients. Recently the General Medical Council – the official body with responsibility for disciplining doctors – suggested that patients might benefit if doctors published information leaflets about their practices and left copies in public libraries. This was a remarkable step into the twentieth century for the GMC, an organization which normally opposes anything which could be construed as 'advertising'.

The idea was welcomed with enthusiasm by just about everyone involved in health care. Except the BMA. The BMA, which knows that such a scheme would benefit patients but might mean that doctors would have to try harder to attract patients by providing better services, opposed the idea.

Fourthly, the BMA has criticized alternative medical practitioners while carefully leaving the field free for doctors. Not long ago the BMA announced publicly that many alternative remedies practised by non-BMA members were of questionable value and contravened the scientific principles of orthodox medicine. A subsequent headline in a medical newspaper was 'BMA beats off the quacks'.

It is interesting to note that there are now said to be over 2,000 doctors in Britain practising 'alternative' medicine. It is fair to assume that many of those 2,000 doctors are members of the BMA.

Fifthly, the BMA isn't always thinking about doctors' careers and earning potential when it makes public statements. Sometimes it is influenced by other things. For example, the BMA recently overturned its own radical policy advocating a ban on all alcohol advertising and promotion and advocated a much more lenient attitude towards alcohol and alcohol manufacturers. You might imagine that this change of heart was inspired by some new evidence showing that alcohol really isn't all that bad for us. Not a bit of it.

The fact is that the BMA had talked itself into a rather tight corner for although it had officially called for a ban on alcohol advertising, the BMA itself runs a Wine Club which exists to sell wine to doctors at specially low prices and to arrange tours to wine-growing areas. Doctors in the BMA had only two alternatives. They could have continued with their own anti-alcohol policy and, to avoid being outrageously hypocritical, have closed their own Wine Club. Or they could keep their Wine Club and abandon attempts to control the abuse of alcohol by banning advertising. The BMA chose the second alternative.

Next, the BMA has undoubtedly got very unhealthy links with the drugs industry.

There are, most independent experts agree, far too many prescription drugs available in Britain. And the confusion caused by all these drugs leads to much unnecessary illness and many unnecessary deaths, because doctors often prescribe products about which they know very little, and because doctors, pharmacists and patients easily become confused by drugs which have similar sounding names, but quite different actions. The proliferation of drugs also leads to higher costs and inadequate testing. But when the Government recently announced that it wanted to force doctors to prescribe some drugs by their chemical names instead of brand names BMA members opposed the idea.

The NHS stood to benefit from the change. And patients stood to lose absolutely nothing. So why did medical spokesmen for the BMA stand shoulder to shoulder with the drug companies in opposition to the Government's plans?

My final protest about the BMA, and the final reason why I think it is doing more harm than good to the British public, is the fact that for many years now the BMA has been campaigning for more doctors. The BMA wants more doctors so that the workload can be spread more thinly. It wants GPs to have a smaller number of patients to look after. But is it in the interests of the public for there to be more doctors available in Britain? I don't think so. And since this is a point that has a great influence on our general health I think it is worth closer scrutiny.

During the last few years, successive governments, influenced by the profession's demands, have made sure that the production of new doctors in Britain has continued to rise. So, for example, the number of GPs in Britain has risen by sixteen per cent since 1978 – an increase that is much faster than the growth in the population. Official policy has been gradually to increase the annual medical school intake towards a target of 4,230. And yet all the evidence suggests that there is a considerable world surplus of doctors. According to recently published World Health Organization figures there are now 45,000 unemployed doctors in Italy and 40,000 unemployed in India. Spain has 23,000 unemployed doctors and the Netherlands has 2,500 without jobs. In Mexico there were 40,000 unemployed doctors in 1984 and in Pakistan 6,000. The Republic of Korea has estimated that by the year 2,000 it will have 26,000 doctors without jobs while Egypt already has 4,000 without work. The United States forecasts an excess of 70,000 doctors by 1990. In Bangladesh recently hundreds of newly qualified but unemployed doctors demonstrated in the streets because they couldn't find work. In the end the police had to make a baton charge to clear them. Even in Britain the BMA itself has admitted that there are 1,500 unemployed doctors. The overall estimate is that by the year 2000 there will be between 250,000 and 500,000 unemployed doctors littering the world's dole queues. And since the number of medical schools has more than doubled in the last ten years things could be even worse than that. Within another fifteen years there could be as many British doctors out of work as there are British doctors in work.

The plain truth is that new doctors are qualifying far more rapidly than existing doctors are retiring. Since it is common for doctors to continue working well into their seventies, eighties and even nineties, the glut of doctors will get dramatically worse with each succeeding generation. By the early part of the twenty-first century the BMA may have real cause to regret its enthusiasm for the training of more medical practitioners. The real tragedy is, of course, that every available scrap of evidence suggests that all these extra doctors do nothing to improve the general health of the population. Theoretically one might imagine that the more doctors there are the better will be the service patients are offered. But there is really no correlation between the number of doctors available and the quality of medical care provided.

One problem is that the cost of paying salaries and fees to all these new doctors means that the limited resources of the NHS are stretched to breaking point.

More important is the fact that the evidence shows that the current excess of doctors merely leads to the over-investigation of simple complaints and the over-treatment of symptoms that would get better without any interference. Dozens of eminent observers within the medical profession have admitted that many medical practices are designed to satisfy the urges and desires of doctors rather than the needs of patients. Dr Mahler, Director General of the World Health Organization, has said that 'the major and most expensive part of medical knowledge as applied today appears to be more for the satisfaction of the health professions than for the benefit of the consumers of health care'. Dr Jonas Salk, famous for his work on polio vaccine, has said that he is 'firmly opposed to the tendency among young physicians to behave primarily as technicians to the detriment of the patient who is treated like an object needing repair'. Not long ago there was a hospital strike in Israel and admissions to hospitals dropped eight-five per cent with only the most urgent cases being admitted at all. Despite this the death rate in Israel was the lowest the nation had ever known. The same thing happened a little later when doctors went on strike in New York City.

If you harbour doubts about all this and you still suspect that the BMA must really know best, let me provide you with some simple but convincing figures.

The consistent argument of those who want to see more doctors in practice is that a better doctor–patient ratio will lead to better health care. That hypothesis is easy to disprove. In America there is one doctor for every 452 people and one hospital bed for every 173 patients. Life expectancy there for white males is 71.8 years. Life expectancy for black males is 65.5 years. In Switzerland there is one doctor for every 816 individuals and one hospital bed for every 177 patients. The average life expectancy for white males is 72.7 years. In France there is one doctor for every 480 people and one hospital bed for every 109 patients. Life expectancy for males is 70.2 years. In Britain there is one doctor for every 1,565 patients (our figures are rather lower than other 'developed' countries, because we don't count doctors in training) and one hospital bed for every 113 patients. Our life expectancy for males is 70.8 years.

Compare those figures to the figures for Jamaica, a relatively under-developed country. In Jamaica there is one doctor for every 7,033 people and one hospital bed for every 360 patients. Life expectancy there for men is 69.2 years.

If you're still not convinced then look at these figures for Korea. In North Korea there is one doctor for every 417 patients and one hospital bed for every 77 patients. Life expectancy there for males is 63 years. In South Korea there is one doctor for every 1,509 people and one hospital bed for every 676 patients. Life expectancy there for males is 64.9 years.

It is clear from all these figures that life expectancy (the most critical and objective assessment of a nation's health) does not depend on the number of doctors in the country. Nor, incidentally, is there any correlation between life expectancy and the number of hospital beds.

The significant conclusion from all this is that increasing the number of doctors is of no medical value. Those members of the medical profession who want to see more doctors in practice in the United Kingdom are working not towards a healthier population but towards a stronger medical profession and shorter working hours.

It seems to me to be clear from all this evidence that the general efforts of the BMA have been designed to improve the lot of its own members rather than to improve the health of the nation. Since the BMA is a trade union this is, perhaps, only to be expected. The pity is that the BMA has been allowed to acquire an authority and a status which gives it far too much control over the organization of health care in Britain.

In the next of my twelve scandals I will describe in some detail the ways in which our surfeit of doctors is harming our health.

SCANDAL No. 2

Ignorance and Incompetence

The second of my twelve scandals, and the second reason why I believe that the health of the nation is getting worse, is the most ironic of all: the fact that through ignorance and incompetence doctors are now themselves injuring patients by the thousand and producing long-term disease problems in epidemic proportions.

As each year goes by, the number of patients injured by doctors increases.

Indeed, medically induced injury is now so commonplace that doctors have a name for it. They call it 'iatrogenesis'.

It is, sadly, one of the fastest growing specialities in modern medicine.

For centuries, critics have claimed that doctors often do more harm than good. Molière, Tolstoy and Shaw all claimed that the average individual would be better off without doctors at all. Sadly, there is now real evidence to show that such an opinion may at last be truly justifable. There is now some basis for the claim that the net value of modern medicine may be a negative one – that by over-treatment, bad treatment and the abuse of technology doctors do more harm than good.

It is difficult to be dogmatic about health and health care but I believe that at least eighty per cent of all patients need no treatment at all and will get better by themselves without any medical intervention. I explained some of the reasons behind this assertion in my book *Bodypower* in which I explained that the human body is equipped with an enormous range of subtle and sophisticated self-healing mechanisms. Of the remaining twenty per cent approximately half need nothing but advice and information. That means that only ten per cent of all patients who are ill genuinely need medical treatment. My claim that the body's internal healing mechanisms are so effective that in at least ninety per cent of illnesses patients can recover without any form of medical treatment has been repeated and quoted many times. My book *Bodypower* has been a bestseller in Britain and in ten other languages and several TV and radio programmes have been based upon its arguments and conclusions. But not one doctor has ever disagreed with this conclusion.

Sadly, however, because both doctors and patients have an exaggerated faith in modern therapies far more than ten per cent of patients receive genuine, aggressive, medical treatment. And that is where the problem really starts because a very hefty percentage of the patients who are treated by doctors are harmed by the treatment they receive. It wouldn't matter so much, of course, if patients were being harmed by treatment they needed . . .

Once again it is difficult to be dogmatic about the number of patients involved, but it has been suggested that in ten per cent of cases medical treatment does positive harm, in another ten per cent of cases medical treatment does nothing at all, and in the other eighty per cent of cases medical treatment does varying amounts of good.

One of the first 'modern' researchers to describe the problems of doctor-induced illness in detail was a doctor called Schimmel who, in 1963, spent eight months studying the patients in a medical ward at Yale University. He showed that 240 of the 1,252 patients there had complications either connected with being in hospital or with the treatments they had received. These complications included reactions to diagnostic procedures, drugs, and blood transfusions as well as infections contracted in the hospital. Forty-eight of the complications were considered serious and sixteen proved fatal.

By 1979 when Steel and his co-workers undertook a five-month statistical study at the Boston University Medical Center they found that 290 out of 815 patients in hospital had suffered some form of iatrogenic (doctor-induced) disease. The 290 patients had a massive total of 497 doctor-induced problems. Serious complications occurred in seventy-six cases and fifteen cases were fatal.

In a study reported in the *New England Journal of Medicine* in 1981 no less than thirty-six per cent of all the patients on a general medical ward of a university hospital had an iatrogenic illness. In nine per cent of these patients the incident threatened life or caused disability. In two per cent of patients the illness was fatal.

Today the problem of iatrogenesis is as bad as ever and affects every patient in Britain who goes near to a general practitioner or a hospital. Speaking at a symposium at the Royal Society of Medicine in London in 1983 Professor Lawson of the Royal Infirmary in Glasgow pointed out that drug treatment side effects occur in no less than twenty-five per cent of patients on medical wards. One of the most dramatic articles dealing with the subject of drug side effects

45

was written by Cedrick R. Martys, a general practitioner from Derbyshire, and published in the *British Medical Journal* in November 1979. In the article, entitled 'Adverse Reactions to Drugs in General Practice', Martys points out that 'of 817 patients in a general practice survey of adverse reactions to drugs, forty-one per cent were thought to have "certainly" or "probably" had a reaction to the drug prescribed. Adverse effects on the gastrointestinal and central nervous systems were the most frequently reported, and ninety per cent of reactions had occurred by the fourth day of treatment'. It seems clear that the doctor-induced illness truly is the fastest growing medical problem in Britain.

Thousands of patients are injured unnecessarily on the operating table and are damaged by incompetently performed diagnostic procedures. Having carefully studied all the available statistics I'm convinced that something like half of all the patients who die on the operating table never needed surgery in the first place while the majority of investigations and tests done in hospital are done for research purposes, as a possible defence against litigation or through laziness. Some of the research papers upon which I have built these conclusions are quoted between pages 61 and 68.

Survey after survey has shown that if you develop fresh symptoms after being treated by your doctor than the chances are that your new symptoms will have been caused by the treatment given to you for your original problems. As I have already said, Dr Martys showed in his paper that forty-one per cent of patients – two out of every five patients – suffer side effects from drugs they are given. And as I've already pointed out if there are ten patients lying in a hospital ward, the chances are that at least one of them will be there solely because he has been made ill by a doctor.

It is the medical profession's unhealthy obsession with drugs which is undoubtedly responsible for a large part of this epidemic of iatrogenic illness. A quarter of a century ago doctors wrote about four prescriptions a year for each of their patients. These days they write out 6.5 prescriptions a head. And the figure is rising. The number of doctor–patient consultations has fallen in the last twenty years but the number of prescriptions has gone up dramatically. In an article entitled 'Are We Overconsuming?' that appeared in the *World Health* magazine recently, Dr Lloyd Christopher of the WHO's Drug Evaluation and Monitoring Unit and Professor James Crooks of the Department of Pharmacology and Therapeutics at the University of Dundee pointed out that in England and Wales the number of prescriptions dispensed by chemists between 1949 and 1964 fluctuated between 188 and 212 million per year. By 1970 the number had risen to 247 million. DHSS figures show that by 1980 doctors were writing out over 300 million prescriptions a year. Not that it is just in the quantity of drugs they prescribe that doctors are at fault. They also prescribe far too many different drugs.

In 1977 the World Health Organization asked a group of experts to decide which drugs were really necessary. The expert committee came to the conclusion that doctors ought to be able to deal with most health problems with a library of 200 drugs and vaccines. Since 1977 the expert committee has reconsidered its list several times, but has made only minor adjustments.

In practice, however, doctors continue to prescribe thousands of drugs that are inappropriate, unnecessary, dangerous or ineffective. So, for example, according to a symposium held at the Royal Society of Medicine in 1983 a massive fifty per cent of the prescriptions written for antibiotics were thought to be quite unnecessary or totally inappropriate. It is important to remember that, useful as they may be, antibiotics can kill. Penicillin alone is said to kill over 1,000 people a year.

One major problem is undoubtedly the appallingly low standard of teaching in Britain's medical schools. Academics are often more concerned with their own research projects than with the students they are paid to teach. The result is that out-of-date philosophies and techniques are handed on to generation after generation and graduates know far too little about the drugs they will spend their lives prescribing.

Similarly, the standard of postgraduate medical education in Britain is extraordinarily low. Most doctors in practice today qualified long before many of the drugs they prescribe were introduced. And yet, as I have already shown, those doctors will have 'learnt' about the drugs they use from drug-company sponsored sources.

Iatrogenesis is not a new problem. Doctors have been injuring people for as long as they have been helping them. Both Hippocrates and Hammurabi recognized the significance of doctor-induced disease. But the epidemic has surely now reached unacceptable levels. It is certainly a major scandal and on the next few pages I will deal with some specific examples.

VARIATIONS IN TREATMENT

In the preface to *The Doctor's Dilemma* playwright George Bernard Shaw points out that during the first great epidemic of influenza, which developed towards the end of the nineteenth century, a London evening newspaper sent a journalist posing as a patient to all the great consultants of the day. The newspaper then published the advice and prescriptions offered by the consultants. The whole proceeding was, almost inevitably, passionately denounced by the medical journals as an unforgivable breach of confidence, but the result was, nevertheless, fascinating: despite the fact that the journalist had complained of exactly the same symptoms to the many different physicians, the prescriptions offered were all different as was the advice he was given.

Nothing has changed. Even in these days of high-technology medicine there are many variations in the treatment schedules preferred by differing doctors. Doctors offer different prescriptions for precisely the same symptoms, they keep their patients in hospital for vastly different lengths of time, and they perform different operations on patients with apparently identical problems.

There are, it seems, no certainties. The unexpected seems to happen so often that it really ought to be expected and the likelihood of a doctor accurately predicting the outcome of a disease is often no more than fifty–fifty. There is ample evidence now available to show that the type of treatment a patient gets when he visits a doctor will depend not so much on the symptoms he describes, but on the doctor he consults.

So, for example, the journal *Modern Medicine* in March 1985 described what happened when 430 Scottish GPs were asked to explain how they would treat a thirty-five-year-old accountant complaining of backache brought on by digging in his garden. The 'case history' was deliberately made fairly precise. Despite this precision, however, the recommended treatments varied enormously. Less than a quarter of the doctors said that they would definitely prescribe a painkiller. Nearly ten per cent said that they hardly ever prescribed a painkiller in such circumstances. Eight per cent of the doctors said they might refer the patient to hospital but fifty-two per cent said they never referred such patients to hospital. Forty-eight per cent said that they usually advised bed rest for up to one week while eight per cent said that they usually advised bed rest for between one and four weeks. Around ten per cent of the doctors said that there was a good chance that they would refer the patient to an osteopath, but the other ninety per cent said that they hardly ever, or never, referred patients to osteopaths. Such enormous differences are surprisingly commonplace these days. Going to a GP really is something of a lottery.

Another survey published in *Modern Medicine*, and this time involving almost 700 GPs in the Midlands, showed that twelve per cent of family doctors might be willing to prescribe a sleeping tablet without even seeing the patient involved. Over half the GPs confessed that they would prescribe a cough medicine without seeing a patient and nearly two-thirds of the doctors said that they might prescribe an antacid without a patient needing to come into the surgery.

A third survey that involved over 400 doctors in Yorkshire showed that one per cent of GPs provide no antenatal care for pregnant women, that forty-nine per cent of GPs never insert intrauterine contraceptive devices in the surgery, that three per cent of GPs do not routinely immunize children and that one per cent of GPs don't provide any contraceptive advice at all.

Despite all these variations in the type of treatment offered most doctors in practice seem to be convinced that their treatment methods are beyond question. Many GPs and hospital doctors announce their decisions as though they are unquestionably correct. On the basis of evidence like this it seems to me that most decisions about how patients could best be treated are based on nothing more scientific than guesswork, personal experience, intuition, and prejudice.

GENERAL PRACTITIONERS ARE LAZY

Every week I get armfuls of letters from readers who want my advice or who want basic, straightforward medical information. A large number of my correspondents apologize for writing to me and go on to say that they don't like to trouble their own family doctor because he is always far too busy. It isn't difficult to see where patients get that impression.

Telephone the average surgery and you'll find that if you want an appointment, you'll have to wait several days; if you want a doctor to visit someone, you'll have to convince the practice receptionist that the only alternative is to wait a couple of hours and call the local undertaker. Once you're in the surgery you'll find yourself being whisked in and out of the consulting room so fast that you wonder why they don't put in a revolving door and save another second or two. All things considered it is hardly surprising that most patients are convinced that British doctors are wildly overworked.

The truth is rather different. Despite this public image, doctors actually spend very little time talking to or dealing with patients. They really are not as busy as they or their patients like to think. Moreover, as the years go by, it seems clear that doctors are spending less and less time seeing patients and making clinical decisions. The number of treatments they initiate is growing rapidly. But the amount of time they spend on initiating those treatments is falling.

I first became aware of this phenomenon when I read an article in *Update* medical magazine written by Dr F. M. Hull, a senior lecturer in General Practice at the University of Birmingham. Dr Hull admitted that when he had examined the way he spent his time, he had been embarrassed to discover just how little time he appeared to work. He was so embarrassed that he then conducted a survey to see how much time other doctors spent working.

According to Dr Hull's figures the average British doctor spends slightly less than twenty-three hours a week talking and listening to patients. And there was even one doctor who admitted to Dr Hull that he spent less than seven hours a week with the patients he was being paid to look after.

Dr Hull wasn't the only doctor to show that GPs are, on the whole, a pretty lazy lot. In 1984 a survey of 199 GPs, conducted by the Department of General Practice DHSS Research Unit in Manchester, revealed that sixteen per cent of GPs spent less than twelve hours a week with their patients, including the time spent on home visits, while only ten per cent spent more than twenty-eight hours with their patients.

What is perhaps most startling about all this is that when the average British GP is compared with colleagues around the world it becomes clear that family doctors in Britain spend far less time with their patients than doctors anywhere else in the world. In Canada, for example, doctors spend twice as much time with their patients. According to a paper that F. M. Hull published in *Update* in 1983 (the paper was entitled 'The GP's Use of Time: An International Comparison') GPs in the United Kingdom spend about twelve per cent of their time with their patients. In the United States of America doctors spend almost fifteen per cent of their time with their patients. In Germany they spend about twenty per cent of their time with patients. And in Canada they spend nearly twenty-five per cent of their time with their patients. It is difficult to avoid the conclusion that British doctors are a pretty lazy lot.

MISTAKES, MISTAKES, AND MORE MISTAKES

For decades doctors have carefully cultivated an aura of infallibility. Occasional errors are accepted as exceptions and excused on the grounds of exhaustion. But for several years now evidence has been accumulating to show that huge numbers of doctors are simply ignorant and incompetent. Here are just some of the recent research studies which have shown the extent of medical ignorance in Britain in the 1980s.

- In *MIMS* magazine in March 1987 it was reported that geriatricians from Gartnavel General Hospital in Glasgow had carried out a study of GP referrals in their area over a one-year period. The hospital consultants had found that the GPs' drug histories were inaccurate in two-thirds of the 700 cases examined. The main fault was that doctors forgot to mention drugs that their patients were taking. For example, the study showed that digoxin, thyroid hormone, and diuretics were not reported in a quarter of the patients who had been prescribed these drugs.

- David Price, a research fellow at the Professorial Medical unit at Leicester Royal Infirmary, studied the records of drug therapy in the hospital notes of patients attending a hospital clinic. Dr Price found that either the hospital or the GP records were inaccurate for more than seventy per cent of the patients. According to Dr Price 'most of the errors were due to patients taking drugs which were not recorded in their notes and some of these errors were potentially serious'.

  Dr Price's study was published in the *British Medical Journal* in 1986.

- In my book *The Medicine Men* (first published in 1975) I reported my surprise at the fact that a number of doctors were still prescribing tetracycline preparations for children. I explained that in the *British National Formulary* in 1971 doctors had been warned that 'all tetracylines tend to delay bone growth and to discolour unerupted teeth'. Way back in 1971 doctors were warned to avoid using tetracyclines in children under the age of seven years.

  In May 1986 the medical newspaper *Pulse* carried details of a report by Dr James Reid (Senior Lecturer/Consultant at the Department of Child Dental Health at Glasgow Dental Hospital and School) and Maura Dunn (Associate Specialist at the Royal Hospital for Sick Children, Yorkhill, Glasgow). Dr Reid was reported to have stated that he still saw children with tetracycline-discoloured teeth and to have estimated that every year thousands of children risk having their teeth ruined because they are prescribed tetracycline preparations. The two dentists issued a plea to doctors not to continue prescribing tetracyclines to young children.

  According to Dr John Wall of the Medical Defence Union, giving children tetracycline products need not necessarily be negligent. He claimed that tetracyclines might occasionally be essential. But many other experts would disagree with him. For example, consultant microbiologist Dr Adrian Bint said in 1981 that, 'It is disturbing that GPs are still prescribing tetracyclines to children. There can be no excuse for this practice since an alternative antibiotic can nearly always be used.'

- In May 1986 the medical newspaper *GP* reported that Dr Badal Pal, Senior Registrar in the Department of Rheumatology at Dryburn Hospital, Durham, had questioned seventy GPs and found that fifty per cent of them knew little about the ingredients of popular non-steroidal anti-inflammatory drugs – probably the most commonly used drugs in medicine today, and taken regularly by millions of arthritis sufferers.

- In July 1984 the Department of Health and Social Security revealed that between January and March 1984 a total of 100 prescriptions had been written and dispensed for four drugs which had previously been withdrawn from the market.

- In November 1984 a survey conducted by the Royal College of General Practitioners showed that many experienced family doctors had inadequate knowledge about the diagnosis and investigation of common disorders.

    Questionnaires were posted to more than 1,400 general practitioners. The questionnaires included questions about common conditions such as anaemia, middle-ear infection, glandular fever, and jaundice. According to Dr William Acheson, Senior Lecturer in General Practice at Manchester University, many of the doctors who responded 'failed to mention answers that were important. Some gave unusual answers and some gave answers that were clearly wrong.' Only half the doctors in the survey mentioned the three most common symptoms in middle-ear infection. More than half left out important questions to ask a patient with jaundice.

    Dr Donald Alastair Donald, Chairman of the Joint Committee for Postgraduate Training in General Practice, said that he was not surprised by the deficiencies revealed in the report. 'All knowledge dissipates at a steady rate unless it is topped up,' he said. 'The average general practitioner spends only four hours a year at postgraduate courses.'

    The average age of the doctors who responded to the survey was forty-six.

- A study of GPs, reported in *Medical News* in January 1982, showed that a quarter of general practitioners do not know of (or do not believe in) the connection between smoking and heart disease. And, according to the survey, twenty per cent of GPs were unaware that cigarettes can cause lung cancer.

It is perhaps interesting, too, to record that in the final examinations for medical students in Paris one-tenth of the candidates made no mention of tobacco when asked to list factors responsible for causing cancer. By contrast thirty-eight per cent of the students mentioned the type of cancer produced in horses' mouths by the rubbing of the bit.

- Writing in the *Postgraduate Medical Journal* in the summer of 1985 pathologists Dr Jane Mercer and Dr Ian Talbot reported that after carrying out 400 post-mortem examinations they had found that in more than half of the patients the wrong diagnosis had been made.

  The two pathologists reported that potentially treatable disease was missed in about thirteen per cent of patients. They also found that sixty-five out of 134 cases of pneumonia went unrecognized while out of fifty-one patients who had suffered heart attacks doctors had failed to diagnose the problem in eighteen cases.

- In September 1986 the Medical Defence Union predicted an epidemic of huge lawsuits resulting from medical blunders. In 1985 the MDU paid out nearly £11.5 million in claims – sixty-five per cent up on 1984.

- In a study reported in the *Journal of the Royal College of General Practitioners* in January 1987 two psychiatrists from Manchester, Professor David Goldberg and Dr Keith Bridges, showed that GPs failed to spot that about half their patients were suffering from psychiatric illness.

- Another report published in the *British Medical Journal* in 1986 showed that attempts to improve the recognition of depression by GPs would be wasted since GPs know little about how to manage depression.

- After withdrawing the pain killer Zomax from the market, the manufacturer Ortho Cilag Pharmaceuticals accused doctors of ignoring prescribing information on drug data sheets. Dr Wendy Jefferson, Ortho's medical director, said that GPs 'should be warned to make sure they read prescribing information correctly'. She added that, 'Since Zomax has been available in the UK, I have had many telephone calls from doctors who have obviously not read the data sheet.'

- A report published in the *Journal of the Royal Society of Medicine* early in 1985 concluded that many hospital patients who suffer heart attacks die during the 'confused and disorganized charades' of attempts to save them because doctors do not know how to give emergency resuscitation.

  According to the report, which surveyed fifty junior doctors at Addenbrooke's Hospital in Cambridge, none of the doctors who took a practical test would have fulfilled a particular set of criteria for effective basic cardiopulmonary resuscitation. Only four of the fifty doctors were able to perform effectively when asked to demonstrate their skills on a model.

  It is also interesting to note that in May 1987 a study published in the *British Medical Journal* showed that when spot checks were done on more than fifty experienced nurses at the Royal Free Hospital in London none of them could give adequate resuscitation in an emergency to patients who collapsed with heart attacks. The nurses were tested on a dummy, without warning, and asked to demonstrate how they would give basic life support to a patient whose heart had stopped beating. The study, carried out by staff from the Cardiology Department and the Psychology Department of the Royal Free Hospital showed that none of the fifty-three nurses tested performed basic life support adequately and thirty of them were assessed as completely ineffective. 'Sisters and charge nurses were significantly more confident than staff nurses,' said the authors of the report. 'In fact, however, they were no more competent.'

  The authors of this report pointed out that in hospital a large proportion of cardiac arrests occur in wards where the nurses have to perform basic life support before the arrival of a team of doctors. The treatment given in the first three or four minutes after a cardiac arrest has a dramatic influence on the chances of survival.

- In February 1987 the Royal College of General Practitioners was so worried about the incompetence of British GPs that it appointed Dr Philip Reilly, Senior Lecturer in General Practice at Queen's University, Belfast, as a 'prescribing fellow' with the special task of investigating GPs' prescribing habits.

  Dr Reilly, who announced that his investigation would last two to three years, said that doctors are often unaware of the degree to which their prescribing varies. 'One doctor might not prescribe anything where others would,' he said. 'The range of medication for arthritis, for instance, is huge and there are many side effects and the use of these drugs is sometimes quite haphazard.'

- In spring 1987 the *Journal of the Royal College of Physicians* contained a report written by Dr David Levy, Consultant Physician at Bolton General Hospital and Professor Michael Lye of the Royal Liverpool Hospital's Geriatric Department which pointed out that many doctors continued to prescribe potassium supplements to patients taking diuretics, even though this practice did far more harm than good.

These are just a few of the specific papers and journal articles which, over recent years, have outlined the inadequacies of modern medical practice and the ignorance and incompetence of many practising doctors. I have quoted these papers at length in order to prove that I am not alone in my fears about the medical profession. I made no extensive search of the medical literature to find these papers.

The main reason for all this incompetence is undoubtedly the fact that for the majority of doctors education stops on qualification. At the age of twenty-five or so a doctor is released upon the community with a head full of fixed, specific knowledge. Two years later doctors are firmly established in practice but their knowledge will be largely out of date. And since the process of undergraduate education is designed to feed information to students, rather than to teach them how to acquire and assess information for themselves, doctors are unable to keep themselves up to date. They are, indeed, vulnerable to those determined to take advantage of their academic innocence for commercial reasons.

Remarkably, there is now ample evidence to show that few doctors make any attempt to keep themselves up to date. In the *British Medical Journal* in February 1987 a report showed that fewer than half of all general practitioners attend any postgraduate education at all. Indeed, the same report also showed that clinical tutors, working in postgraduate medical centres, devoted very little of their time to education – most doing two hours or less a week.

The result is that by the time doctors are forty years of age or more they will probably be dangerously out of date. The forty-year-old doctor will have qualified and finished formal medical training long before the introduction of many of the drugs he or she commonly prescribes. He will have left medical school long before surgeons started doing transplant operations and long before CAT scanners became widely available. He may have attended a few drug company sponsored lectures and he may have had lunch with a few drug company representatives. He will certainly have been bombarded with drug company literature. But he is fairly unlikely to own any up-to-date medical textbooks or to read regularly any journals that are not paid for or subsidized by the drug industry. I doubt if one doctor in ten ever reads anything about medicine that isn't either paid for or subsidized by the drug industry.

And if forty-year-old doctors are out of touch, then what about fifty-year-old doctors? And what about Britain's 500 doctors who are over the age of seventy? There are, believe it or not, many doctors in Britain who qualified before penicillin became available. Many of these doctors know absolutely nothing about the majority of drugs they use except what they have been told by the companies making and selling those drugs.

Finally, an example which further demonstrates that doctors are just as prone to making mistakes as any other members of our society. In March 1987 the *British Medical Journal* published the results of the 1987–1988 BMA council elections. Voting doctors handed in a grand total of 16,118 ballot papers. Of those no less than sixty-one papers were 'spoilt'. In other words one in every 264 doctors couldn't even put an 'X' in the right place. It is hardly surprising, therefore, that doctors often make mistakes when writing out prescriptions, making diagnoses or writing letters to one another.

PRESCRIBED DRUGS – AN ENDURING PROBLEM

The explosion in the number of available prescription drugs has been causing concern for many years now. Back in 1961 Dr Walter Modell of Cornell University Medical College, one of America's foremost drug experts, wrote in *Clinical Pharmacology and Therapeutics* asking, 'When will they [doctors and drug companies] realize that there are too many drugs?' He went on to point out that there were then 150,000 preparations in use of which seventy-five per cent did not exist a mere ten years previously. He added that about 15,000 new mixtures and dosages hit the market each year, while only about 12,000 died off. 'We simply don't have enough diseases to go round,' he lamented. 'At the moment the most helpful contribution is the new drug to counteract the untoward effects of other new drugs.'

Since 1961 the position has continued to get worse. By the late 1970s the world's trade in legal drugs was growing at fourteen per cent a year and the manufacture and marketing of drugs had become a multi-billion-pound industry. Today most drug experts readily agree that doctors prescribe far too many pills and potions and that extremely serious problems are produced by this endemic overpre-scribing. Almost inevitably, therefore, the incidence of drug side effects has also reached endemic proportions.

In Britain there is now ample evidence to prove that two out of every five patients given pills by a doctor will develop side effects – usually within four days of starting their treatment. Some side effects are fairly mild – a rash or a little diarrhoea, for example. But a considerable number of patients suffer troublesome and often harmful side effects from prescribed drugs.

Amazingly the evidence now shows that if there are ten people in a hospital ward then the chances are that one of those patients is in hospital because he has been injured by prescription drugs. Life threatening or not, side effects are now so common that if you develop a new set of symptoms while taking pills your doctor has prescribed, the chances are that your new symptoms were caused by your treatment.

There are many reasons for the size of Britain's growing prescription drug problem. The drugs industry must, of course, take some of the blame. For years now many companies have shown a callous disregard for the welfare of patients and a distinct preference for profits. It is difficult to ignore the suspicion that drug companies enthusiastically produce new products for profitable long-term conditions such as arthritis and high blood pressure and then cynically withdraw them and replace the drugs when accumulating side effects begin to cause controversy – and threaten the company with possible lawsuits. In two of my previous books, *The Medicine Men* and *Paper Doctors*, I outlined in detail many of the dishonest practices espoused by the drugs industry.

But I don't believe that the drugs industry should take all the blame for all our current problems with prescription drugs. Three other groups of people should also share the responsibility: patients, doctors, and the controlling authorities.

First, patients. It may sound strange to insist that patients should take some of the blame but there are sound reasons for this suggestion. In the past patients have often put too much faith in drug therapy and have pushed doctors into over-prescribing. I don't think it is true today, but ten or twenty years ago it was undoubtedly a fact that doctors felt under an obligation to prescribe because they knew that patients leaving their surgeries without a prescription would be disappointed.

In addition patients must take some of the blame for problems which develop because they have ignored instructions given to them when the drugs were prescribed. A survey published in the *British Medical Journal* early in 1987 showed that most patients are given very specific instructions on how to take their drugs. But other surveys have shown that many patients fail to follow the instructions they are given. For example, Mr John Sharp, a project manager of the

Association of the British Pharmaceutical Industry told an audience of 1,000 pharmacists attending a conference in Jersey in September 1986 that 'between thirty and fifty per cent of British patients, some of whom are seriously ill, do not comply with prescribers' instructions'.

Modern drugs are extremely powerful and have to be taken properly if side effects are to be kept to a minimum. A drug designed to be taken at eight-hourly intervals must be taken at eight-hourly intervals and not just three times a day. If a doctor tells a patient to take pills in the morning, then the pills should be taken in the morning and not at midday or in the evening. The human body changes continually throughout each twenty-four-hour period and many drugs have a different effect at different times of day. For example, one tablet of hydrochlorothiazide taken as a diuretic in the afternoon will have a fifty per cent greater effect than if taken in the morning. The antihistamine effect of a drug called cyproheptadine lasts for seven hours if taken at seven o'clock at night but for sixteen hours if taken at seven o'clock in the morning.

Patients also often forget that some drugs don't mix well with certain foods. Drugs such as indomethacin should never be taken on an empty stomach while monoamine oxidase inhibitors can kill if taken together with cheese, game, yeast extracts, or certain wines.

The doctors' share of the blame for our prescription drug problems is their failure as a profession to understand just how dangerous drugs can be and just how important it is to keep drug use down to an absolute minimum. Indeed, rather than trying to curb their enthusiasm for prescribing the majority of doctors actually spend time and effort working out ways to enable them to prescribe more drugs with less effort.

One of the biggest problems of all is 'repeat prescribing' which has now become standard practice for the majority of doctors. Every single day of the working week half a million repeat prescriptions are collected from GPs' surgeries – that is one-half of all the prescriptions that doctors write. Back in 1979 J. G. R. Howie, writing in the second edition of the Royal College of General Practitioners' *Trends in General Practice*, pointed out that fifty per cent of prescriptions were issued 'without direct doctor–patient contact'.

Like many bad habits repeat prescribing was started for sensible reasons. The original idea was to benefit patients suffering from long-term disorders, such as diabetes, who didn't need regular monthly examinations, but who did need to pick up prescriptions regularly for their drugs.

What started off as a sound and sensible way to save time has become one of the major causes of illness in Britain today. Pills that may have been necessary once are now provided automatically without any check to see whether or not they are doing any good – let alone any harm. Millions of patients have been taking pills they don't need for years. Every day people are made ill – or even killed – by drugs that they never really needed to take.

Repeat prescribing is now such an important part of medical life that in some practices extra receptionists are employed to do little else but write out prescriptions for doctors to sign. I've even known doctors pre-sign prescription forms and then allow untrained staff members to fill them in afterwards when patients say what drugs they want.

Read through the medical journals these days and you will see that there are many articles about repeat prescribing. But the majority of these articles are not critical – they simply explain how to make the practice more efficient. In the journal *GP* in April 1985 Dr Graham Hunter, a GP practising in East Sussex, wrote an article entitled 'How to make repeat prescribing easier' in which he openly admitted to signing 1,500 prescriptions per month – a staggering 18,000 per year. Justifying his argument that issuing a year's supply of tablets at one go might not be a bad idea, he pointed out that writing out 18,000 prescriptions on a monthly basis would take him a solid 1,500 hours of work, but if he wrote out annual prescriptions for his patients, the chore would take only 125 hours.

Perhaps the most remarkable indictment of the 'repeat-prescribing' phenomenon was the £500 fine an unnamed GP in Bradford was ordered to pay in February 1986 for continuing to issue repeat prescriptions for a patient who had died.

In the days when drugs were as harmless as they were ineffective repeat prescribing would not have mattered much. Today all pre-scribed drugs are powerful and potentially dangerous. Repeat pre-scribing is a dangerous practice.

The drugs industry, patients, and doctors must all share some of the blame for the overuse of drugs and the problems that develop as a result of that overuse. But the regulatory bodies which exist to protect us from potentially dangerous drugs and drug-prescribing practices are also culpable.

In Britain the Government's official drug watchdog – the body responsible for keeping dangerous drugs off the market and for ensuring that drugs are used properly and safely – is the Committee on Safety of Medicines. It was the thalidomide tragedy that originally inspired the development of a drug watchdog in Britain, and the first such body was the Committee on Safety of Drugs which was set up in 1963. In 1971, the same year that the Medicines Act became law, the Committee on Safety of Medicines replaced it.

The Committee on Safety of Medicines is the most important of the Government's advisory committees and it has a number of specific functions. According to the Medicines Act the CSM has the responsibility for scrutinizing new drugs before they are tried clinically, for scrutinizing drugs after they have been tested and before they are marketed, and for keeping a watch on drugs after they have been marketed. It is one of the CSM's most important roles to monitor adverse reactions and to warn doctors about possible drug problems. Technically the CSM has no legal authority, but because it is an advisory committee to the Government (appointed, not elected), it does, in practice, have a considerable amount of power.

Sadly, however, in its short history the CSM has shown itself to be either remarkably incompetent or remarkably uncaring. It is neither good at spotting problems early on nor is it good at dealing with problems once they have been defined. There are several reasons why it is a failure.

First, the CSM is far too slow to pick up evidence of drug problems. The twenty doctors and pharmacists who comprise the Committee on Safety of Medicines are supported by over 100 full-time doctors, pharmacists and lawyers, and backed up by a host of administrators and a nationwide network of 150 part-time medical officers. But despite this huge professional staff the CSM still relies heavily upon reports from GPs who are invited to fill in yellow cards when they notice a side effect or dangerous drug reaction. In theory completed yellow cards should provide the CSM with a constant supply of warning information. But the system falls down because most doctors don't bother to make reports. Between 1972 and 1980, for example, eighty per cent of doctors eligible to complete yellow-card reports did not report any side effects associated with any of the drugs they had prescribed.

Estimates vary but my research shows that at best one in twenty-five drug reactions will be reported – so for every twenty-five patients who suffer severe problems with a prescription drug only one doctor will actually make an official report. Professor William Asscher, Chairman of the CSM, told a meeting in London in June 1987 that doctors are slovenly about reporting side effects. He estimated that still only ten to fifteen per cent of adverse reactions were reported. That is the CSM's first problem: it just doesn't have access to the basic information it really needs.

The second problem is a much more serious indictment of those who run the CSM. Even when it does have the information it needs, the CSM is far too slow to respond. The CSM's short history is littered with examples of prevarication and delay.

It was so slow to act over the drug practolol (one of the early beta-blockers) that the company making it brought in controls voluntarily before the CSM had made a move. Marketed in 1970, practolol (known also by the brand name Eraldin) was prescribed largely for the relief of angina and high blood pressure. Only after being used for four years was it found that practolol could cause a bizarre syndrome involving dangerous damage to skin, eyes, ears, and intestines.

The anti-arthritis drug Opren was only withdrawn from the market in 1982, nine months after doctors had warned the CSM of severe problems. By the time action was taken the CSM had received reports linking the drug to 3,500 serious side effects and over sixty deaths.

Although the drug is no longer available, the manufacturers are contesting patients' claims for damages.

PROBLEMS IN THE OPERATING THEATRE

So far in this chapter I have dealt mainly with the sort of incompetent professional behaviour displayed by physicians and, in particular, by GPs. To restore the balance a little I now want to concentrate on surgeons who are, as a group, unbelievably inefficient and very inclined to follow their own individual philosophies rather than acknowledged therapies.

There are a number of specific problem areas worth highlighting. Firstly, because they are allowed to do as they like, surgeons working in the NHS are inclined to follow their own rules. If car workers at a factory in the north of England took twice as long to produce a car as workers in a factory in the south of England eyebrows would be raised, time and motion experts would be called in, and questions asked by indignant shareholders. But that is exactly the sort of discrepancy that exists within the NHS.

One surgeon will keep a tonsillectomy patient in hospital for six days while another surgeon with an identical case will send his patient home after twenty-four hours. Obviously, the first surgeon will have a longer waiting list than the second.

This sort of variation in efficiency doesn't just add to the length of NHS waiting lists and the cost of running the health service, it also contributes to the amount of post-surgical illness patients have to endure. There is evidence to show that long-stay patients will take longer to recover and that patients who get out of hospital quickly stand a much better chance of getting better without complications. Patients who stay in hospital longer than necessary run a variety of risks. They are likely to undergo tests and investigations that they don't really need (this hazard is described in greater detail on pages 73 to 78); they are likely to suffer from anxiety, sleeplessness and malnutrition and they run an increased risk of developing some sort of infection. So, for example, in 1981 Dr Peter Meers, Deputy Director of the Public Health Laboratory Service, reporting on the first national survey for 120 years of the risks faced by hospital patients revealed that nearly one hospital patient in ten develops an infection after admission. Other experts have shown that infections acquired in hospital can be particularly difficult to treat since the causative organisms are often resistant to antibiotics.

Surgeons get away with this incompetence by claiming that all patients are different and that it is impossible to generalize when dealing with the human body. That excuse only stands up for individual cases. It does not excuse surgeons whose patients' average hospital stay is prolonged. And there is plenty of solid evidence to show that huge differences do exist.

In a paper published in the *Journal of the Royal Society of Medicine* in August 1985 Dr Nick Black of the University of Oxford wrote that a 'study of geographical variations in the rate of surgery for glue ear reveals striking differences between both English health regions and health districts. There are twofold differences between regions and up to sevenfold differences between districts. Analysis of these differences at different levels of population aggregation reveals that professional uncertainty about the indications and value of surgery for this condition is the major factor responsible.'

Similar variations have been shown for hysterectomies, gall-bladder removal and tonsillectomy. It is difficult to find any logical scientific reasons for such differences.

Another general problem is that a great many surgeons are 'knife happy' – they are far too ready to operate on their patients even when surgery isn't necessarily the best solution to a patient's problems.

In a paper called 'Overtreatment in Surgery' which was read to the Section of Surgery of the Royal Society of Medicine on 5 December 1984, Dr F. G. R. Fowkes, Senior Lecturer in Epidemiology at the University of Wales' College of Medicine, said that 'examples of overtreatment abound in every surgical speciality and occur to varying degrees with almost every operation.' Dr Fowkes, who supported his claim with twenty-four scientific references, argued that if through research and expert consensus better clinical guidelines for surgical intervention could be developed and implemented, fewer unnecessary operations would be performed.

Dr Fowkes is by no means the only observer to believe that surgeons perform too many operations. The *Drug and Therapeutics Bulletin* (published by the Consumers' Association) has reported that 20,000 appendix operations are performed unnecessarily each year in Britain. In 1982 Sir George Godber, Chief Medical Officer at the Department of Health and Social Security, wrote that, 'it is commonly believed that many of the 90,000 tonsillectomies done in England and Wales are of questionable benefit.'

Why are so many unnecessary operations performed? One widely acknowledged argument is that many of the patients having tonsillectomies and other common operations are treated privately. Others are put on to NHS lists in order to keep those waiting times as long as possible. People do not want private operations unless the health service list is a long one.

If you think that sounds cynical, consider another popular operation that brings in a good income for many surgeons and which is also done far more often than is necessary: the operation performed for the treatment of patients with peptic ulceration. I would argue that many of the patients with this particular problem would benefit from a solution or medication taken from outside the traditional, narrow avenue of possibilities. But surgeons have the choice of a safer, non-surgical alternative which many prefer to ignore for their own commercial reasons. There is, in fact, a drug available called cimetidine which has been shown to heal seventy-five per cent of duodenal ulcers in four weeks and a further ten per cent in eight weeks. It has been estimated that by its use the number of operations could easily be cut by up to half.

More evidence to suggest that some surgeons may over-operate on their patients is provided by the National Association of Health Authorities in Britain which has shown that while some surgeons do less than 150 operations a year, other surgeons do more than 750 operations a year.

Apart from the pain and inconvenience patients have to go through when having unnecessary surgery, there are very real risks to be considered.

There are approximately 2.2 million surgical operations and procedures performed each year in England. That is about five operations for every 100 potential patients. Normally there is a one per cent fatality record associated with surgery (although this figure rises to sixteen per cent for routine operations performed on ninety-year-old patients) and if thousands of patients are having unnecessary surgery then thousands are dying unnecessarily. For example, if just ten per cent of the operations performed each year are unnecessary, then surgeons kill 2,200 patients a year quite unneccesarily.

(This figure is not 'plucked out of the air'. The maths is simple and straightforward. If we take the lowest 'average' mortality figure and assume that one per cent of the 2.2 million surgical operations performed each year result in death there will be 22,000 deaths associated with surgery. If ten per cent of operations are unnecessary, it is fair to assume that ten per cent of the deaths are unnecessary too.)

In addition, of course, there are other lesser risks to be taken into consideration. Complications after surgery are fairly commonplace. In a report published in the *Journal of the Royal Society of Medicine* in June 1984 Mr A. Pollock of Scarborough Hospital reported that in a study of some 1,200 laparotomy operations (operations in which the abdomen is cut open) he had found some sort of post-operative complication in forty-seven per cent of the operations.

To put the evidence I've cited into proper perspective I should point out that in my opinion approximately one-half of all surgical operations and procedures are unnecessary. That means that surgeons murder 10,000 people a year and produce a horrifying amount of unnecessary mutilation and suffering.

Surgeons, of course, have a number of clever defences to accusations of over-treatment. No patient can prove that an operation was unnecessary if he has an operation done. But if a patient doesn't have an operation and survives, then the surgeon can simply say that he was lucky. If the patient doesn't have an operation and dies, then the surgeon has proved his point. Looking back through history surgeons have nearly always operated and have nearly always harmed patients unnecessarily. Today things are no better than they ever were.

To further illustrate my claim that surgeons operate unnecessarily I have chosen three specific types of surgery.

First, coronary artery surgery. This particular type of surgery is especially interesting because in recent years the DHSS has made great attempts to increase the number of operations done. In 1978 a modest 3,200 coronary artery bypass operations were carried out in Britain. In 1983 over 9,400 coronary artery bypass operations were performed. This figure seems likely to rise fairly rapidly and most British heart surgeons would like to see the number of operations performed multiplied several times. (Perhaps they would like to see their departments become larger and more powerful.) To accommodate the surgeons the DHSS has recommended that coronary artery bypass surgery should get priority when health authorities are working out their budgets.

When it was first introduced just under two decades ago bypass surgery was hailed as the biggest medical breakthrough for decades.

The aim of it is, as the name suggests, to provide an alternative route for blood around fat-clogged arteries. Heart attacks are often produced when arteries become clogged and fresh, oxygen-carrying blood supplies can't get through. Surgeons performing the bypass operation either use artificial material to construct new arteries or else they use the patient's own leg veins.

Almost inevitably, since heart disease, which kills between 150,000 and 180,000 people each year in Britain alone, is the greatest killer of our time, bypass surgery has become extremely popular. In America coronary bypass grafting operations are now extremely common – over 100,000 such procedures a year being performed as long ago as 1980.

But there is one big problem with the coronary bypass operation: there has never been any real evidence to show that it is worth doing. Indeed, a number of observers have argued that coronary bypass operations are dangerous and useless. A massive Coronary Artery Surgery Study performed in the United States showed no difference between medical and surgical treatment as far as many patients were concerned. Other studies showed that over a ten-year period approximately half the patients who have surgery will develop heart pain again. It seems that the younger the patient the less successful the operation is.

In July 1985 the *Medical Journal of Australia* published an article by Richard F. Heller and Stephen R. Leeder pointing out that although the enthusiasm there for performing coronary artery bypass surgery was increasing, the most recent trials have failed to show a significant overall survival benefit from surgery. The authors suggested that other approaches (including lifestyle advice and medical treatment) could be more effective as well as being less expensive.

The only really large clinical trial that has so far been conducted to measure the efficiency of coronary artery surgery was the Veterans' Administration report that was published in the late 1970s and which showed that medically treated patients had a three-year survival rate of eighty-seven per cent while those who underwent surgery had a survival rate of eighty-eight per cent.

But life expectancy isn't the only way to measure the success and usefulness of an operation, of course. A bypass operation takes several hours to perform and involves a lengthy stay in hospital. It can be an exhausting and debilitating experience for a patient. It can, and often does, prove lethal. Many experts now readily admit that there is a one in thirty risk that a patient undergoing coronary artery bypass surgery will be dead within thirty days of the operation. Although mortality figures vary from centre to centre and surgeon to surgeon, a mortality rate of two per cent is very good and the mortality rate can be ten times as high as that. Anything up to a quarter of patients having the operation have heart attacks either while on the operating table or shortly afterwards. (If you want to read review articles summarizing the available evidence I suggest an article entitled 'The outlook for patients after coronary artery surgery', written by the Irish surgeon T. Aherne and published in *Modern Medicine* in March 1987 and a paper written by C. J. Hilton, a consultant cardiothoracic surgeon from Newcastle, writing in *Update* in October 1981.)

In May 1987 a report in the *Quarterly Journal of Medicine* concluded that, 'Many patients who have cardiac surgery end up worse off after the operation than before it because their quality of life has been impoverished.'

Recognizing that coronary artery surgery (now the most common procedure performed in cardiac surgery) has been in use for nearly thirty years without anyone trying to find out how patients' everyday lives are affected by the operation, doctors at Oxford's Warneford Hospital carried out a 'quality of life' survey. Dr Richard Mayou reported that some patients lived in constant fear of death while others worried about how long the operation would be effective for.

When asked to comment on the study for the doctors' newspaper *Pulse*, Dr Celia Oakley, Consultant Cardiologist at Hammersmith Hospital, said that she found the results disturbing. One of the most startling facts to emerge from the study was that whereas nearly half of the patients who had had the operation had been working right up to the time of surgery, three months after the operation only just over a third of the men were working. And a year after the operation nearly half the patients were still not working – despite the fact that according to Dr Oakley even manual workers should be back at work by three months after a coronary bypass operation.

However, none of the gloomy evidence has stopped surgeons performing this operation. And, apart from the clinical trials I have mentioned, there have been no attempts made to assess the value of the operation. Responding to pressure from surgeons the DHSS has committed itself, and NHS resources, to an operation that seems certain to do more harm than good.

So much for coronary artery bypass surgery. The second type of surgery that is commonly done despite the fact that there is no evidence to show its value is surgery for obesity. Perhaps I should rephrase that: there is no evidence to show that surgery for obesity is effective *and* safe.

For a number of years now surgeons have been performing operations on overweight patients. One of the operations most commonly performed has been intestinal bypass surgery which involves – as the name suggests – bypassing a huge length of intestine. First pioneered in the 1960s by surgeons in Los Angeles this operation has been performed fairly frequently in Britain by R. M. Baddeley, a consultant surgeon at the General Hospital in Birmingham. According to Baddeley a series of 220 patients over a period of five years lost, on average, thirty-five per cent of their original body weight. But consider the side effects. Baddeley himself admits that the side effects associated with the operation (performed, remember, to help patients lose weight) are potentially numerous and require vigilance on the part of the responsible clinician.

There are three main groups of complications: the metabolic problems produced by diarrhoea and malabsorption; changes in the liver and malnutrition produced by the fact that the body does not absorb the nutrients it needs; and the effects of bacteria moving into the small bowel. Baddeley says that excessive diarrhoea (more than five watery stools a day) can result in potassium, magnesium, and calcium depletion. He also says that this need not occur if patients limit themselves to between 1200 and 1500 mls of fluid a day. They should, he says, suck ice if they feel thirsty.

Patients also stand a good chance of developing kidney stones and forty-two per cent of patients develop pains similar to rheumatoid arthritis in their small joints. Cirrhosis, vitamin deficiencies, wasting, neurasthenia, foul flatus, and tuberculosis are just some of the other problems known to be associated with this operation.

The third type of surgery that I want to deal with specifically is breast surgery for cancer. Since the beginning of this century the standard operation for breast cancer has been the mastectomy. Sometimes the operation has been a simple removal of the breast itself (a simple mastectomy) and sometimes it has involved more extensive mutilation in which flesh, muscles, skin, and lymph nodes are all removed (a radical or extended mastectomy). Naturally, women who have the second, more disfiguring operation suffer more than women who have the simple mastectomy. But women who have a mastectomy of any kind suffer personal, social, and mental distress far greater than women who have less extensive surgery.

Over the last few decades many studies have confirmed that in the vast majority of cases radical mastectomies may be unnecessary. For example, in a study that was later published in the *New England Journal of Medicine*, Dr Umberto Veronesi and his colleagues at Italy's National Cancer Institute followed 701 women with small breast tumours between 1973 and 1980. About half of the women had radical mastectomies while the rest lost only a quarter of their breasts. The results showed no difference between the two groups and the researchers commented that radical mastectomy seemed to involve unnecessary mutilation.

In the *British Medical Journal* in 1979, a paper described results obtained after studying 3,878 women with breast cancer between 1954 and 1964. The authors of this paper, Allan O. Langlands and Gillian R. Kerr of the Department of Radiotherapy at Edinburgh Royal Infirmary and Western General Hospital, Stuart J. Pocock of the Department of Clinical Epidemiology and Social Medicine at the Royal Free Hospital in London and Sheila M. Gore of the Department of Statistics at the University of Aberdeen, concluded that 'treatment by simple mastectomy and radiotherapy is generally accepted to give results equivalent to more radical surgery'.

In October 1986 the *British Medical Journal* contained a report of the Second King's Fund Forum at which a panel of doctors agreed that 'there is no evidence that mastectomy or more extensive surgery, as opposed to local removal of the tumour, leads to longer survival'.

By late 1986 most experts around the world were agreed that the majority of women with breast cancer did not need to have their breasts removed at all.

And yet despite all this evidence some surgeons have continued to perform radical mastectomies. It is difficult to avoid the conclusion that such surgeons must be either callous and indifferent or stupid and ill-read.

In April 1987 Mr Ian Fentiman, Consultant Surgeon at Guys Hospital in London, took the unusual step of criticizing other surgeons when he announced to the annual meeting of the Cancer Research Fund that breast cancer is not well treated in Britain. 'Treatment which conserves the breast is suitable for the majority of women but the majority of women are not getting it,' said Mr Fentiman, who estimated that eighty per cent of women with breast cancer could be successfully treated without the need for a disfiguring mastectomy.

Despite all this evidence, and despite the fact that a five-year study of women with cancer has shown that a patient's attitude has a very important part to play in deciding whether or not she survives, thousands of women are still having their breasts severed and their lives devastated by surgeons.

SCANDAL No. 3

High Technology

There is, of course, no inherent scandal in the development of high-technology medicine. In principle any advance which improves the ability of doctors to diagnose and treat ill health must be considered an advantage.

But problems do arise with high-technology medicine because too many doctors regard the technology as the end rather than the means. Medicine is the most applied of all applied sciences but in recent years the search for new technology has often become an end in itself. Too many doctors practising medicine have forgotten that their primary aim should be to preserve and restore good health. The problem for many doctors is that the scientific medium has become more important than the humanitarian message. I am by no means the only doctor to have noticed (and been appalled by) this tendency. Dr Jonas Salk, famous for his work on the polio vaccine, has said, 'I am firmly opposed to the tendency among young physicians to behave primarily as technicians, to the detriment of the patient who is treated like an object needing repair.'

In hospitals and clinics all over the country there are now doctors who see (or who practise as though they see) artificial hearts, CAT scanners and intensive-care equipment as ends in themselves. The old joke that the operation was a success, but the patient died, is no longer much of a joke.

High-technology medicine should be the icing on our health-care cake. The tragedy is that too many doctors are making icing and not enough doctors are baking cakes.

I trained as a doctor in the late 1960s and can still vividly remember many of the lessons I learnt as I walked the wards as a medical student. I can, for example, clearly remember a patient called Mr Wills.

Mr Wills was the father of one of the ward sisters and when he was brought into the teaching hospital where I was doing my training he looked readier for the mortuary than a hospital bed. He was in his mid-seventies and it was so difficult to tell whether he was alive or

69

dead that the nurse who accompanied him to his bed immediately put out a cardiac-arrest call. It was an impressive entrance to the ward.

Mr Wills was a chronic asthmatic and the victim of two previous heart attacks. It was difficult to tell whether his pulmonary dysfunction was making his heart worse, or whether his failing heart was contributing to his pulmonary dysfunction. In addition there was the problem of ensuring that the pills given to alleviate the symptoms of his heart condition did not exacerbate his lung trouble, and vice versa.

Within minutes of his arrival on the ward Mr Wills had one tube down his throat and another in one of his veins. He had an oxygen mask strapped across his mouth and a catheter in his bladder.

Stimulating drugs had been injected into a vein in the back of one of his hands and a urine-collecting bottle, in practice an opaque plastic bag, had been pinned to his bedclothes.

After about an hour or so Mr Wills woke up, began to breathe a little more easily and started to look more like a patient and less like a cadaver. Three hours after his admission he collapsed again. A team of doctors and nurses worked through the night to keep him alive. At nine o'clock the next morning Mr Wills was conscious, although only just, and that ungodly hound Cerberus had been kept at bay only by a series of dramatic interventions.

At eleven that same morning Mr Wills collapsed again, this time having a heart attack and disappearing from the land of the living with the stealth of an experienced burglar. With much ado and many electrical aids he was dragged back again. At this time I began to suspect that Mr Wills was no longer a willing partner in these heroic endeavours.

By late afternoon Mr Wills' cheeks were hollow, his eyes dark and seemingly bottomless and he looked, quite literally, like death warmed up. Which is what, I suppose, he was. He had, two specialists agreed, almost certainly suffered severe brain damage during one tussle with death. No one could tell for certain what damage had been done because for hours Mr Wills had remained marooned half-way between consciousness and unconsciousness.

That evening I sat with him while his daughter, our ward sister, took a brief rest. For a moment Mr Wills opened his eyes, saw me sitting alone and with an effort that brought beads of sweat to his brow, shook his head from side to side. His eyes caught mine and even in my innocence I felt that they were the eyes of a man who knows there is no hope, knows that he must die and wants only to die quietly, quickly, and painlessly. Mr Wills, I realized, had come to

70

terms with death. The trouble was that no one else had come to terms with his death. Guiltily, I looked away.

Twice that night he died again and twice he was brought unceremoniously back to life. The electrocardiograph machine which stood constant guard on his bedside locker provided instant warning of impending doom. At each interruption of his heartbeat the alarm would sound and Mr Wills would be rescued once more.

All attention on the ward was on the curtain drawn around his bed. It seemed as though every piece of electrical equipment in the hospital was now stored in that small space. The other patients were unusually quiet and depressed. Mr Wills served as a constant, ever-present reminder of their potential fate. Each time he disappeared into a world beyond life they waited nervously, as if they feared that they might disappear with him.

Mr Wills died during the eighth attempt to resuscitate him. He died at seven in the morning with a tube down his throat, a tube in his urethra connecting his bladder to a plastic bag, a needle in each arm and one in his leg, a pair of defibrillating paddles by his side, a smear of grease on his chest, a scatter of broken vials and torn cellophane envelopes on his abdomen, an oxygen mask on his face, an electrocardiograph machine on his locker, a long cardiac needle in his heart, a smear of blood on his cheek and a puddle of spilt drip fluid under his bed. He died lying on the floor with his arm in the puddle and his pyjama trousers round his ankles, his pyjama jacket ripped, and his hair damp with sweat. He died despite or because of our attentions and he died without dignity or peace.

When I left I heard his daughter, Sister Wills, talking to her mother in the corridor outside. 'We did our best for him, Mother,' I heard Sister Wills whisper as she sipped a cup of tea. And although at the time I didn't really understand my doubts I couldn't help wondering if she was right; had we really done our best for him, or had we done our best for us? That was, I suspect, the first time that I realized that high-technology medicine isn't always in the patient's interest.

While still a medical student I had come face to face with the fact that the aims and ambitions of those practising high-technology medicine do not always coincide with the aims and ambitions of individual patients. Later I was to discover that there are two other major problems associated with high-technology medicine. First, buying, developing and using high-technology medicine often takes up huge resources, and the sort of heavy expenditure involved may be quite inappropriate. Secondly, high-technology equipment is itself often used inappropriately. I'll deal with these problems in the pages which follow, but first I should define what I mean by high-technology medicine and some of the specific aims of those who practise high-technology medicine.

The easiest way to describe high-technology medicine is 'complex, expensive and, inevitably, restricted in availability'. By and large just about anything with a plug on the end of it is a piece of high-technology equipment though there are, of course, within this definition many grades of high technology.

Naturally, all those who practise high-technology medicine believe that they have the interests of their patients at heart. Sadly, however, many of them are technicians who are more interested in pure science than in seeing patients walk away from hospital in good health.

To the modern specialist high-technology equipment means many things. Surrounded by the latest equipment he feels comfortable, professional, secure, and powerful. The modern specialist acquires status and professional standing from the equipment he has available to him. Over the years I have met and spoken to many consultants who have admitted to me privately that acquiring the latest piece of expensive equipment is in many ways no different to acquiring the latest model motor car. The consultant's personal strength will often be based on the number of impressive machines he has at his command.

By and large patients are confused by it all. There are many who have an implicit faith in any new technology. These patients always prefer to be tested by the latest equipment and they feel slightly cheated if they aren't plugged into an incomprehensible-looking machine that is covered with dials and flashing lights. But others are less convinced by it all. They are unhappy with the mechanization of modern medicine. They yearn for the older, simpler days. These patients prefer the human touch and they feel uncomfortable, frightened, and alone when abandoned to the impersonal modern equipment.

These patients are well aware that there is now a very real risk that doctors will dedicate themselves to looking after the machines and leave the machines to do the task of looking after the patients. And their fears are justified. In the past doctors used machines to give credibility to their decisions. Today, however, patients are beginning to feel uncomfortable about letting computers make 'life and death' decisions.

In addition patients are becoming more and more aware that machine-inspired or machine-aided intervention will often be wasteful and irrational. Consider another true anecdote. Again this comes from my days as a medical student.

George Taylor was eighty years old when I first met him on a porter's trolley in a casualty department. I was working alongside a young casualty officer, trying to gain experience at the sharp end of hospital practice. Mr Taylor had fallen in his terraced home where he lived alone and he had banged his head on a table. There was a small cut and a little blood, but the main problem was that Mr Taylor had lost consciousness.

The young casualty officer wasn't sure what to do and so he called the surgical registrar. The surgical registrar wasn't sure what to do either and so he arranged for our patient to be taken to another department for a CAT scan of his head. Working in a teaching hospital these facilities were readily available.

When Mr Taylor came back to the casualty department, the CAT scan report showed that he had some bleeding inside his skull. Having found a specific lesion, the registrar had no option but to call in a consultant neurosurgeon. The nearest on-duty neurosurgeon was thirty miles away but he arrived at the hospital within an hour.

Naturally, the neurosurgeon decided to operate. Four hours later the operation was over and Mr Taylor was occupying the last available bed in the hospital's intensive-care unit. Technically he had 'died' twice, but the neurosurgeon wasn't keen to have his records marred by a death on the operating table and so he encouraged the anaesthetist to keep the patient alive artificially.

A week later Mr Taylor was still in the intensive-care unit. He still hadn't regained consciousness and there was no sign that he ever would. The problem here had been that no one had been willing to take the responsibility not to use the high-technology equipment that was available. And an eighty-year-old man had been subjected to a series of complicated and extremely expensive procedures not because they were necessary or suitable, but because they were available. And that is, perhaps, the major problem with high-technology medicine: those with access to this type of sophisticated intervention-ism still aren't sure just when the application of their equipment will be appropriate.

In the rest of this chapter I will deal in detail with some specific aspects of high-technology medicine.

TESTS AND INVESTIGATIONS

After studying dozens of scientific papers on the subject, talking to scores of hospital doctors and GPs and spending over ten years practising medicine within the NHS I am convinced that at least two-thirds of all tests and investigations ordered by doctors are unnecessary. Every year thousands of doctors practise blunderbuss therapy and order huge numbers of unnecessary tests.

A hundred years ago there were hardly any diagnostic tests available. Then the only hazard was that a doctor would 'overtreat' his patients. Today a doctor can choose from thousands of individual tests and overinvestigation probably leads to even more problems than overtreatment. Unnecessary tests can be misleading, time consuming, painful, expensive, and dangerous. In 1980 J. A. Stilwell and two colleagues wrote an article entitled 'Evaluation of Laboratory Tests in Hospitals' (which was published in the *Annals of Clinical Biochemistry*). They confirmed that many tests were requested thoughtlessly, wasting resources. In 1979, in an article entitled 'Cost of Unnecessary Tests' in the *British Medical Journal*, Sandler showed that the routine examination of blood and urine contributed to only one per cent of the diagnoses made. In June 1987 in an article entitled 'Are Routine Bacteriological Cultures Necessary in an Accident and Emergency Department?', published in the *British Medical Journal*, Drs Hashemi and Merlin from the Accident and Emergency Department at Walsall General Hospital in the West Midlands produced some startling figures. They pointed out that 'microbiology services receive many requests that cannot reasonably be expected to influence management of patients.' Their study was designed to evaluate the usefulness of taking bacteriological swabs in the accident and emergency department of a district general hospital. Their conclusion was that 'routine sampling for microbiological testing is unnecessary.' Astonishingly they reported that in only three per cent of cases was the treatment given based on the result of culture and antibiotic sensitivity. Moreover, they pointed out that in over sixty per cent of cases the patient was discharged before the results of culture were available.

Doctors overinvestigate their patients for a number of reasons. First, overinvestigation is a habit that doctors are taught when young. Young students and newly qualified doctors are encouraged by consultants to order all the available tests as though they were getting special wholesale rates. Consultants encourage this behaviour by criticizing students mercilessly for not ordering as many tests as can possibly be done. No thought is given to the cost of all these investigations, no attempt is made to decide which tests are particularly likely to help doctors reach a diagnosis, and no thought is given to the patient who will spend hours and days wandering from laboratory to X-ray department and will end up exhausted and exsanguinated.

Secondly, doctors order tests in order to impress their students, their colleagues, their patients or themselves. The more esoteric the test the greater the status associated with its use.

Thirdly, doctors frequently order unnecessary tests because they are planning to write papers for scientific journals and because they need lots of data to fill up their pages and help build up their reputations. Most of the papers published in this way are of little or no genuine clinical value.

Fourthly, tests are sometimes performed in order to protect doctors from the risk of litigation. So, for example, doctors in hospital casualty departments will frequently order unnecessary X-rays in order to protect themselves against any possible accusation of negligence. Occasionally, there is some slight justification for this nervousness. On the whole, however, this fear is misplaced.

Fifthly, many doctors practice 'hot' or aggressive medicine and insist on collecting all the possible evidence they can even when the diagnosis is not in doubt. So, for example, this type of doctor will insist on performing an endoscopy so that he can actually see a stomach ulcer even though the patient's history and the barium-meal examination have both made the diagnosis impossible to avoid.

Sixthly, unnecessary tests are often ordered to buy doctors time when they don't know what is going on. They hide behind technology and seek reassurance and comfort from more and more new tests. The condition of the patient becomes almost irrelevant as they search for that ever-elusive diagnosis.

Finally, many doctors perform unnecessary tests simply and solely because that's how it's always done. So, for example, patients who are in hospital will often have daily blood tests even though there is absolutely no need for daily blood results and even though a daily change in the results obtained is unlikely to lead to a daily change in the treatment provided. In other words investigation and diagnosis have been completely divorced from treatment!

There are, of course, a number of hazards associated with this fetish for overinvestigation. One of the most important anxieties I have is that tests and investigations are often extremely dangerous. Not surprisingly, perhaps, relatively few scientific papers have been published describing the dangers associated with hospital tests but there have been some papers published and some figures are available.

For example, in a paper entitled 'Frequency and Morbidity of Invasive Procedures', published in the *Archives of Internal Medicine* in December 1978, three physicians from the Departments of Medicine at the University of California and Stanford University showed that fourteen per cent of all patients who underwent invasive procedures (such as biopsies, catheterizations or bronchoscopies) had at least one complication. Most complications then need treatment and involve a longer stay in hospital for the patient.

Even patients who have been to hospital and had simple basic blood tests will know that occasionally things can go wrong. Sometimes the problem is simply an escape of blood into the tissues with the development of a painful swelling. But sometimes more serious problems can develop. Arteries can be punctured or nerves can be hit accidentally. The majority of doctors (and nurses) regard blood letting as a trivial task. In fact it is painful, expensive, and potentially dangerous. And, more often than not, unnecessary.

The second big problem with investigations is that they often produce 'false positives'. In other words although patients do not have a particular disease a test may show, wrongly, that they do have that disease. The consequences of this vary.

When the first blood test for syphilis was introduced doctors accepted it as accurate. It wasn't until several decades later that doctors found that fifty per cent of all the patients whose blood test had shown them to have syphilis didn't have syphilis at all. The lives of many of those patients must have been ruined quite unnecessarily. It is particularly poignant to note that eighty-five per cent of patients who do get syphilis but who are untreated will have an entirely normal life span and seventy per cent of such patients will have no evidence of the disease when they die.

Sadly, the available evidence suggests that most doctors still don't understand the significance of obtaining false positives.

In April 1979 the *Lancet* published a paper entitled 'The Value of Diagnostic Tests' which reported that when doctors and medical students were asked to interpret a simple statistical problem most of them got it badly wrong. The question was: 'If a test to detect a disease, whose prevalance is one in 1,000, has a false positive rate of five per cent, what is the chance that a person found to have a positive result actually has the disease?' Out of sixty professionals who were asked this question twenty-seven answered ninety-five per cent while eighteen answered two per cent.

This means that little more than a quarter of those questioned understood the principles of basic statistics. The correct answer should have been that one person out of the 1,000 can be assumed to have the disease. Therefore 999 people will not have the disease, but five per cent of these, or roughly fifty, will give a false positive result. Consequently only one out of fifty-one people with a positive result will actually have the disease.

This sort of statistical analysis of investigations may seem to be only of academic value. But in practice such anomalies are extremely important.

Most doctors regard laboratory tests as invariably accurate. When the results come back from the laboratory, they are regarded with the sort of reverence once accorded to messages on tablets of stone. But the plain fact is that most laboratory tests are only ninety-five per cent accurate – even when all the equipment in the laboratory is working absolutely perfectly (something that usually happens about once a week). As a general rule ninety per cent accuracy is more likely. So, if a patient has twenty laboratory tests done (a figure that is probably fairly accurate these days) then the chances are that even if he is perfectly healthy the tests will show at least one abnormality. And that is when the trouble starts.

When doctors spot an abnormality then they think in terms of disease. And when they think of disease they think in terms of treatment. The treatment involved will, of course, depend upon the false positive that has been obtained. But from this simple example it is easy to see that just about every patient going into hospital will have a good chance of being treated for a disease he hasn't got. Indeed, simply having the diagnosis made can sometimes change a patient's life. One recent study showed that out of ninety-three children who had been diagnosed as having heart disease – and who had lived as 'heart patients' – only seventeen really had heart disease.

So far in this chapter I've dealt largely with laboratory tests and investigations. But ever since Rontgen first discovered X-rays at the end of the nineteenth century radiology has played an increasingly important part in the average doctor's investigative armamentarium. Go into hospital for a fairly routine operation and there is an excellent chance that they'll take at least one X-ray – even if it's only a routine X-ray of your chest.

How much good do all these X-rays do? The answer, I'm afraid, is that most of them are entirely unnecessary. They are potentially hazardous, they are extremely expensive and they are extremely unlikely to contribute anything to your doctor's knowledge of your illness.

One of the first papers to have been published criticizing the number of X-rays done appeared in the *British Medical Journal* in November 1968 when a radiologist and a neurologist estimated that the consumption of X-ray film was doubling every thirteen years. Dr J. W. D. Bull and Dr K. J. Kilkha concluded that their study gave 'ample evidence that the great majority of plain X-ray films taken for such conditions as migraine and headache, did not contribute materially to the diagnosis.' They pointed out that much time and effort was wasted by doctors, radiographers, and patients. Their plea for doctors to think before ordering X-rays fell on deaf ears.

In 1975 the *British Medical Journal* again printed an appeal for doctors to order fewer X-ray pictures. By then it was estimated that the number of radiological examinations was increasing by ten per cent every year. This time the report in the *BMJ* pointed out that after routine X-rays were taken of 521 patients under the age of twenty not one serious abnormality was detected. In all these patients chest X-rays were taken.

Once again doctors were asked to order fewer routine X-rays. Once again the appeal was ignored.

By 1983 the problem had become such an important one (and such an international one) that the World Health Organization issued a statement saying that 'routine X-ray examinations frequently are not worthwhile. Doctors,' said the WHO, 'ask for X-rays as a comforting ritual.' The WHO report went on to point out that X-rays are so overused and misused that they constitute a major source of population exposure to manmade ionizing radiation. It also pointed out that X-rays account for between six per cent and ten per cent of a country's expenditure on health.

Since something like ninety per cent of all X-rays are unnecessary it is clear that between five per cent and nine per cent of Britain's expenditure on the NHS could be saved simply by finding some way to stop doctors ordering useless X-rays.

But the evidence suggests that little has changed and that doctors are still wasting just as much time, money, and energy as ever. In March 1987, for example, Nottingham medical school lecturer Dr Jim McCracken reported on a study he had co-ordinated into the treatment of pneumonia in general practice. McCracken concluded that it simply is not worth carrying out routine X-rays on recovered patients who have no clinical abnormality. It seems unlikely that this report will have any greater effect on the number of unnecessary X-rays being ordered than did the report written by Professor James Bull back in 1968.

SCANNERS

Scanners should, you might suppose, appear in with X-rays and other forms of tests and investigations. They are, after all, merely an extremely sophisticated way of finding out what is going on inside the body. But for a number of reasons I believe that scanners are rather special. They cost far more than any other form of investigative equipment. They are regarded – both by patients and doctors – with more awe than any other form of investigative equipment. And they are misused more often.

In my view scanners' use in Britain today is a perfect example of the unacceptable face of high-technology investigative medicine. There is nothing wrong with scanners themselves – it is the way in which they are used and abused that is a scandal. But before I go on to explain why I think scanners are wrongly used I will first explain what they are and how they work.

It was back in the late 1960s that scientists first started to experiment with computed tomographic scanning (CT scanning for short). Scanning cleverly combines radiological and computer techniques in order to produce a series of cross-sectional pictures of the head or the body. In principle the technique is fairly simple: X-rays are passed through a cross-section of the body and detected on the other side. As with conventional X-rays the difference in intensity between the X-rays entering and leaving the body depends upon the intensity of the intervening tissues. The computer helps take hundreds of thousands of separate pictures – building these up into a cross-sectional picture.

Although research had been going on in this field in several parts of the world, it was at EMI's research laboratories in Britain that the first CT scanner was devised – and the first patients to be scanned, in 1971, were British.

CT scanners have two main advantages over conventional radiology. First, the technique is more sensitive than conventional radiology and can pick up smaller lesions. Secondly, because of the three-dimensional pictures that are built up structures and lesions within the body can be viewed even though they would normally be obscured by overlying tissues. In theory, therefore, scanners have a great deal to offer.

However, I don't think these machines are quite as wonderful or as worthwhile as they might seem to be. The first words of caution about these machines appeared in the *Lancet* in November 1974 when an editorial writer pointed out the danger of the scanner being overused. Pointing out that X-rays and other investigations are commonly overused by doctors, the writer of the editorial suggested that we needed to take great care in the deployment of these machines. With scanners, he explained, the risks of overuse are the same, but since the machines are so expensive to buy and to run, the stakes are considerably higher.

By the late 1970s scanners were becoming extremely popular and many other authors were beginning to ask questions about their value as clinical tools.

For example, in America, where 800 scanners had been installed by 1979, the National Academy of Science's Institute of Medicine called for an evaluation of this extremely expensive diagnostic technique. The Institute questioned the wisdom of devoting an ever-increasing slice of inevitably limited resources to the purchase of equipment that had not even been shown to be of clinical value. One of the major problems spotted by the Institute was the fact that many of the conditions diagnosed with the aid of a scanner were untreatable. When the scanner finds a small tumour hidden away from normal X-rays, the doctors involved can make a neat and precise diagnosis – but they can do nothing about the disease.

In January 1979 the *Journal of the American Medical Association* reported that the Public Health Service in America had published guidelines regulating the purchase of CT scanners in an effort to prevent 'the unnecessary proliferation of this useful but expensive new technology'.

The same issue of *JAMA* also included details of a thirty-three-month study that had taken place at the Veterans' Administration Hospital and the University of California Medical Center in San Francisco. Drs Christopher Baker and Lawrence Way assessed the value of CT scans in 202 randomly selected cases. This was one of the very first proper clinical trials of scanners.

The authors acknowledged that their data verified CT scans as technically impressive and often providing anatomical detail that would otherwise be unavailable, but concluded that 'in our experience CT scans were of great help in a few cases and were very misleading in others, with the majority having a marginal impact, either positive or negative. In this last group, consisting of seventy-eight per cent of all the scans, patient management would not have been appreciably changed if the CT scan had not been performed.'

Another study, also reported in *JAMA* in 1979, was designed by radiologists at the Massachusetts General Hospital in Boston, USA, who wanted to find out how computed tomography affected both diagnoses and treatments. According to this study 'in almost half the cases the answers could be interpreted as positive in that results of a CT scan led to a change in diagnosis. Influence of the scan on therapy, however, was not marked.' The Boston team showed that in general physicians found that the CT scanner had no influence on the treatment offered to patients.

These studies startled many doctors who had thought that scanners really did promise much. And although radiologists using scanners attempted to show the value of this new equipment, all the published evidence seemed to support the depressing conclusion that scanners had no practical role to play in modern medicine.

In 1982 the *Lancet* published a paper entitled 'Is Routine Computerized Axial Tomography in Epilepsy Worthwhile?' The paper was written by four doctors working at the Departments of Neurology and Neuroradiology at Salford Royal Hospital. The answer to their question was a fairly resounding *no*. The authors concluded that 'careful clinical assessment and examination supported by an electroencephalogram remain of paramount importance in the management of epilepsy.'

In 1985 the *Scottish Medical Journal* published a paper entitled 'Chronic Subdural Haematoma in the CT Scan Era' written by a team of doctors and surgeons from Glasgow. These experts concluded: 'One hundred and fifty patients with chronic subdural haematomata were studied with respect to clinical features, investigation and outcome. The outcome in this series of patients, managed after CT scanning became the standard method of investigation, was no better than in previous studies.' The authors finished by pointing out that CT scanning does not result in improved results in patients with subdural haematoma.

There were, of course, a few spirited attempts to defy the growing feeling that CT scanners had no real value. Two neuroradiologists and a neurologist from Frenchay Hospital in Bristol wrote a paper in the *BMJ* in 1983 entitled: 'Computed Tomography in the Investigation of Dementia'. These three authors found that ten per cent of all the patients who had been examined with the scanner had a treatable lesion and they concluded that 'if a few patients with treatable lesions can be identified then the benefits to all concerned may be incalculable.'

But a closer examination of the facts suggests to me that the authors had not really approached their task in a truly objective and critical manner. They did not, for example, compare the usefulness of the scanner with other (and possibly far cheaper) ways of reaching an accurate diagnosis. And they did not question the significance of the information obtained with the aid of the scanner.

Out of the 500 patients they examined, four who had tumours survived for an average of twenty-one months. The average age of these patients was seventy-three, but three of these patients had no treatment. It seems to me perfectly possible that clinical examination of these patients, together with traditional diagnostic techniques, would have identified most of the lesions.

As evidence accumulated to show that CT scanners are of doubtful value so those who control the NHS purse strings started to show more and more reluctance to purchase scanners. These are, after all, incredibly expensive pieces of equipment to buy and to run. An average sort of scanner will cost at least £500,000 to buy and tens of thousands of pounds to run. At a conservative estimate the cost per patient per scan is £200.

But NHS radiologists weren't pleased by the decision to cut down on these machines. To the professional diagnostician the CT scanner is an essential piece of equipment: it gives him status among other radiologists and it inevitably enlarges the size and budget of his department. It is also a fascinating piece of equipment to operate. Depriving a radiologist of the latest piece of equipment is like expecting a Grand Prix driver to go out on to the track in last year's car. And so for years now radiologists have led local fund-raising schemes designed to find the cash to buy a local scanner.

It isn't difficult to see why these fund-raising schemes are successful. The doctors who organize the appeals usually argue that a scanner is the latest and most efficient piece of diagnostic equipment available; they argue that the local hospital should have such a piece of equipment and that without an appeal local patients will be deprived of access to such machinery. And the doctors organizing these appeals can usually find a small child whose life has been saved with the aid of a scanner. Fund-raising is done in a very emotive way. No one bothers to point out that the child would probably have been saved anyway. And no one bothers to point out that the cost of running the scanner will probably take vast sums of money out of the hospital's limited resources.

The result is that within a few months or a year or two enough money will have been raised to buy a scanner. The local radiologist will once again be able to raise his head among his peers. His department will have the latest piece of machinery installed.

In spring 1987 I asked the DHSS in London to tell me just how many of Britain's scanners have been bought in this way and 'given' to local hospitals to run. The answer staggered me. In the 1970s a total of thirty-seven head scanners were purchased and twelve are still operational (scanners have an even shorter working life than motor cars – they are abandoned not when they stop working, but when they are superseded by new models). And so far a total of about 160 body scanners have been bought – and 150 of these are still operational. About forty-five per cent of all these scanners were bought wholly or partly by voluntary fund-raising activities. Such appeals are still commonplace today.

Nearly half of all the scanners in Britain were bought to satisfy the professional egos of a few radiologists rather than to satisfy genuine local needs. I firmly believe that the evidence now proves that in those hospitals where scanner appeals have been successful the standard of medical care provided will have declined as a direct result of scanners being bought. When an appeal fund donates a scanner to a hospital it leaves the hospital to pay the running costs of the machine. According to the DHSS the cost of running just one scanner is now approximately £100,000 a year. Inevitably, this means that other parts of the hospital will have to be deprived of resources. Wards will have to close, waiting lists will get longer, nurses will not be replaced and standard, essential, life-saving equipment will remain in use long after its natural lifespan has been exceeded. And, of course, when a new model scanner comes on to the market in a couple of years' time the radiologist will want his 'old' scanner replacing. He will either persuade the hospital to update his already unnecessary equipment or he will merely launch another local appeal to raise the necessary funds.

INTENSIVE-CARE UNITS

For thirty years now intensive-care units or coronary-care units have been regarded as essential centres in all large, general hospitals. The principle behind the special-care unit is an old one. Back in 1852 Florence Nightingale wrote that 'it is valuable to have one place in the hospital where postoperative and other patients needing close attention can be watched.' And today the availability of modern, sophisticated monitoring equipment means that the intensive-care unit can be given a very impressive appearance. Few physicians would dare to suggest that the hospital should abandon the idea of preserving a special unit within the hospital where severely ill patients can be cared for.

In some hospitals the unit is intended for any patients who need close attention, in other hospitals the unit is primarily intended for patients who have had heart attacks, and in very large hospitals there may even be two units – one for patients who need intensive care and one for patients who have had coronaries.

These units are filled with high-technology equipment. They are shrines to modern electronics and computer technology. But are they really useful? Do they have a role to play in keeping patients alive? Or are they just another example of technological waste? Are they another example of high technology for the sake of high technology?

Let's take a look at the evidence. The first important point is probably the most obvious. Patients don't go into intensive care for specialized treatment. They don't even go into intensive care for specialized nursing care. Patients are admitted to intensive-care units or coronary-care units for close observation. The idea is that the patient who is in one of these units can be monitored carefully and consistently for any change in his condition. Then, if a problem develops, treatment can be applied.

So, the obvious questions are: how useful is this observation and does it save lives? The answers are that it doesn't seem to be very useful and it doesn't seem to save lives.

A study done at the Massachusetts General Hospital between 1977 and 1979 showed that out of 2,693 patients admitted to an intensive-care unit, observation resulted in treatment being required in only ten per cent of the cases. And a paper published in the *Journal of the American Medical Association* in December 1981 and written by doctors from the Intensive-Care Unit Research Unit and the Departments of Anaesthesiology and Clinical Engineering at the George Washington University produced similar results, showing that eighty-six per cent of all the patients admitted to an intensive-care unit did not require any treatment. These two research studies clearly suggest that the majority of patients who go into intensive care cannot be critically ill since they don't need any treatment.

It also seems fairly clear that if no treatment is necessary then being in the intensive-care unit can't really save many lives. Again the available evidence supports this conclusion.

Over the last few years a number of studies have startled the medical profession by their demonstration that putting a patient into an intensive-care unit or coronary-care unit does not improve that patient's chances. For example, in May 1987 a paper entitled 'Mortality From Myocardial Infarction in Different Types of Hospitals' appeared in the *British Medical Journal*. Written by a team of eminent physicians this paper showed that patients actually stood a better chance of staying alive in a simple cottage hospital than in a sophisticated coronary-care unit in a large teaching hospital. The team also showed that even when patients needed resuscitation they stood just as good a chance in a country hospital as they did in a large teaching hospital. The authors concluded that 'the results of this study should suggest to both health administrators and clinicians that increased resources for coronary care, either for new services or for upgrading existing services, may not be required.'

Other studies have shown that patients stand just as good a chance of surviving after a heart attack if they stay in their own homes as they would if they went into a special unit. (See page 6.)

It must seem inexplicable that a patient who has a heart attack and goes into a specialist coronary-care unit has a poorer chance of surviving than a patient who just goes on to an ordinary hospital ward. How can that possibly be?

The answer, of course, is that intensive-care units and coronary-care units are, for a number of quite specific reasons, very dangerous places. The high-technology shrine is no place for a vulnerable, easily damaged, sensitive human being.

The first problem is that the patient who goes into a coronary-care unit will be treated like a battery hen. He will be tied up to a row of frightening machines and deprived of all contact with the real world. Instead of comfort, sympathy and understanding, he will be surrounded by cold, clinical, computerized efficiency. The intensive-care unit is designed for doctors, not patients. It is a perfect breeding ground for research papers. It is a terrible place for a sick patient.

In January 1985 the coronary-care unit at the 800-bed Charing Cross Hospital in London had to close after Dr Peter Nixon, one of the pioneers of specialized coronary-care units, announced that patients who went into the unit were being frightened to death. 'Patients put into a coronary-care unit enter a strange new world,' said Nixon. 'Wired up to monitors and flashing lights, their autonomy is completely removed. They are subordinated to a system of machinery and people in white coats who may not talk to them very much that they don't understand and have no means of controlling. Going through one of these units creates conditions that might increase the risk of a heart attack.' Nixon also said that when he put patients under hypnosis he had found that even the recollection of being in a coronary-care unit could start a heart beating abnormally.

Many other doctors have commented on the psychological problems produced in a coronary-care unit by the ever-present bleeping, flashing, and ringing machinery. Patients can't sleep, they can't relax and they are treated like idiots. It is hardly surprising that at a Consensus Development Conference on Critical Care Medicine held at the National Institutes of Health in America in March 1983 it was agreed that anxiety and psychiatric disturbances are common complications produced by being in an intensive-care unit.

Important though it undoubtedly is, fear is not, however, the only problem patients have to face when they go into one of these high-technology units.

The second major danger is that patients in these units may be harmed by the procedures being used to observe them. While in an intensive-care unit a patient will probably be subjected to a host of investigative and monitoring procedures.

For example, when repeated blood samples are required a catheter may be placed inside the radial artery. Three studies have shown that up to fifty per cent of patients suffer serious complications when this is done. (Two of the studies were published in the journal *Anaesthesiology* in 1983 the other was published in the *British Journal of Anaesthesia* in 1977.) Cardiac catheterization, another common but usually unnecessary investigation in which a tube is pushed into the heart in order to measure its efficiency, is also very dangerous. Indeed, a number of patients who undergo this investigation will die as a direct result. Coronary angiography, a test which involves injecting a contrast medium into the heart and then taking a series of X-rays, also kills a number of patients.

To these problems must be added the fact that diagnostic errors and investigative errors are as common in intensive-care units as they are in other hospital departments. It is perhaps hardly surprising that patients who spend time in such units have nightmares. According to Dr D. W. Ryan, Consultant Clinical Physiologist and Consultant in Administrative Charge of the General Intensive Therapy Unit at the Freeman Hospital, Newcastle upon Tyne, writing in a July 1986 edition of the medical journal *Update*, between ten and twenty per cent of patients who are admitted to intensive-care units continue to have hallucinations and unpleasant dreams or recollections after leaving the unit.

Intensive-care units and coronary-care units cost a great deal of money to run – at least £1,000 per patient per week. In March 1987 details of a multicentre study entitled 'How Do Physicians Adapt When the Coronary Care Unit is Full?' were published in the *Journal of the American Medical Association*. To show how physicians adapt to limited CCU beds the authors compared what happened to patients when beds were available in CCUs and what happened when CCUs were full and beds were not available. The conclusion was that 'physicians can safely adapt to substantial reductions in the availability of CCU beds'.

PREGNANT WOMEN AND BABIES

During the late 1960s high-technology medicine started to have a strong hold over the field of obstetrics. Pregnancy and childbirth – natural and often trouble-free processes – were taken over by the technicians.

In 1970, following the recommendations of the Peel Committee, it became national policy to encourage all mothers-to-be to have their babies in hospital. According to the Peel Committee, having babies in hospital would reduce the risks in childbirth both for mothers and for babies.

But most of the members of the Peel Committee were themselves hospital obstetricians or midwives. They either ignored or didn't understand the fact that most of the young mothers and babies who were dying during childbirth came from lower social groups. They took no account of the fact that if money had been spent on providing better maternity grants, better antenatal care and better back-up facilities, the result would almost certainly have been a reduction in mortality rates. The hospital-based consultants on the Peel Committee had a vested interest in increasing the expenditure on hospital-based facilities and so the facilities for home births were dramatically reduced while the amount of money available for high-technology medicine increased rapidly.

As the 1970s went by, it became ever clearer that this decision had been a disastrous one.

In hospital in the early 1970s electronic foetal monitoring had been introduced and suddenly the very natural business of giving birth became a very complicated business. Suddenly there were reports that births were being induced and that huge numbers of women were having Caesarean sections rather than being allowed to deliver their babies in the normal fashion. High-technology medicine had taken over childbirth.

The results were fairly disastrous. Thousands of women began to complain that having a baby was no longer enjoyable. There were many objections raised about women being artificially induced to give birth at times convenient for the doctors and midwives. And there was even evidence to show that forcing women to have their babies in hospital was not clinically sound. As I pointed out in my book *Paper Doctors* (published in 1977 by Temple Smith), Holland had a lower infant mortality rate than Britain and yet two-thirds of Dutch women had their babies at home without the help of ultrasound, amniocentesis, epidural anaesthesia, pelvic arteriography and a dozen other complicated, expensive, and dangerous procedures. In 1976 a doctors' conference in New York came to the conclusion that it was safer for women to have their babies at home since high-priced intervention will needlessly damage between ten and fifteen per cent of children born in hospital.

Not only did women not like having their babies in hospital, but the evidence showed that they were better off having babies at home – away from interfering doctors and midwives.

Nor was it only mothers who stood to gain by having their babies at home. There was also evidence to suggest that babies were better off at home, too.

During the 1970s the increasing interference in the natural processes of childbirth had been matched by an increase in the amount of high-technology medicine being used to care for newly born babies. There was, in particular, a proliferation in the number of special baby-care units. In 1964 a modest 6.2 per cent of all newly born babies were admitted to special baby-care units. By 1975 a massive 18.4 per cent of newly born babies were being taken away from their mothers and put into special units. Most of the babies being admitted to special units were not admitted because they needed help or support, they were admitted because the units were there. Mothers were being deprived of their babies and babies were being deprived of their mothers for no sound clinical reason at all.

The available evidence showed that this enforced separation of mother from child was not merely unnecessary and unpleasant, it was also positively harmful. An editorial in the *Lancet* in March 1979 concluded that 'the overall suggestion from the published work is that the degree of early physical mother–infant contact – perhaps even in the first hours after birth – may affect the mother's confidence, mode of handling, and duration of breast feeding and even the intellectual and motor development of the child. These differences are more clearly defined in infants whose separation is prolonged.' The editorial writer went on to point out that when mothers and babies were separated there was an increased risk of baby battering, cot death, and an unexplained failure to thrive.

By the early 1980s there was a huge amount of evidence available to show that the artificial constraints favoured by obstetricians and midwives often did pregnant women and their babies more harm than good. Obstetricians, once among the most popular of all specialists, had become widely hated and despised by women.

In 1982 a working party appointed by the Royal College of Obstetricians and Gynaecologists came to the conclusion that 'a flexible attitude on the part of medical and midwifery staff to antenatal and intrapartum care and a willingness to consider alternative approaches as ideas change is essential to maintain the confidence of pregnant women.' Coming just ten years after the Peel Committee had led the profession directly into the world of high technology this was a remarkable statement.

But this apparent about-turn by Britain's obstetricians was more of a public-relations job than a genuine attempt to improve things. The report acknowledged the fact that there is a need to balance the hazards of invasive, interventionist procedures against their benefits, but it also stated unambiguously that all births should be in hospital!

It is, therefore, perhaps not particularly surprising that today things are much the same as they were in the 1970s. Women and their babies are still exposed to far too much high technology. The only real hope for the future comes from the fact that there is now an overwhelming amount of evidence to show that all this interference makes things worse rather than better.

The only question is, how much longer will Britain's obstetricians and midwives continue to put their faith in a style of high-technology medicine that has now been discredited?

THE ULTIMATE ARROGANCE

For some years practising doctors have designed their working day not around the requirements of the patients they see but around the capabilities of the high-technology equipment at their disposal. The equipment is not there to help them heal their patients; the patients are there to help them use, and justify, the equipment.

Now, in the last year or two, there have been signs that some doctors are no longer satisfied with this modern variation on their traditional rule. Many surgeons and physicians in practice today would prefer to use their skills and their technology to help them fulfil a more fundamental role. Traditionally medicine is practised to try and maintain the laws of nature and repair faults which may develop. Today, however, a growing number of practitioners are becoming Faustian in their attempts to circumvent the laws of nature by using technology to help them rewrite the rules. Unwilling to accept nature as the ultimate decision-maker these doctors are attempting to improve on the design of the human body and to make fundamental alterations which will enable us to live longer, healthier lives. Instead of devoting their time to repair work a growing number of doctors are now anxious to go into the design business.

So far I have discovered three examples of this latest trend in the worship of high-technology medicine; three examples of an arrogance and an impertinence which does not fit easily or comfortably within the traditional confines of medical care.

Leaving aside the fact that I find this approach offensive and outrageous, what also disturbs me is that I strongly suspect that in the long run it will enable tomorrow's scientists to do even more harm than their predecessors.

The first example comes from the world of surgery. As I have already explained in this chapter, surgical treatment for breast cancer has kept thousands of surgeons busy for a considerable number of years. Today, however, there are surgeons who would like to take surgical intervention one stage further: they want to remove breasts *before* the cancer develops.

So far these surgeons, operating mainly in America, have removed breasts from over 10,000 women who had no cancer and no other illnesses. In each case the surgeon has removed the breast tissue and replaced it with a silicon-filled plastic bag. The aim of the surgery has been to eradicate the risk of cancer developing. However, there is no evidence to show that this brutal form of preventive medicine does actually stop cancer developing.

The other two examples involve drug treatment. The first is the suggestion that we should all take regular doses of daily aspirin in order to help us avoid developing heart disease. According to those researchers who recommend this potentially hazardous activity, people who take regular doses of aspirin are less likely to develop blood clots. And the theory is that if we all take our daily aspirin, we will be less likely to have strokes and heart attacks.

I see this form of intervention as potentially very dangerous. How can any scientist be sure that long-term dosage with aspirin won't irritate the body in some way? And how can we be sure that by changing the way in which our blood clots form we are not leaving ourselves open to other circulatory problems? Finally, what about the risks associated with the normal use of aspirin? There is, it seems to me, a genuine risk that anyone following this line of treatment will simply die of stomach ulceration instead of heart disease.

The other suggestion is that in order to avoid developing breast cancer women should take regular doses of a powerful anti-cancer drug called tamoxifen. Here the theory is based on the observation that tamoxifen interferes with the balance of the natural female hormones oestrogen and progesterone. The problem is that naturally occurring female hormones help protect women from heart disease. So how do the scientists know that their suggestion won't prevent one disease while making another more likely? The answer is that they don't. Nor is there any guarantee that by changing the way in which the body is constituted we will not damage future generations.

Having studied the contributions made to our lifestyle by high-technology medicine I feel that we should, perhaps, show a little more humility. We still know very little about how the human body works. We still know very little about how to keep ourselves healthy. We are still vulnerable to a whole host of potential hazards.

Surely it is absurd that we should try to make fundamental changes to the basic design of the human body when all the available evidence shows that our attempts to devise and use new forms of high-technology medicine have been remarkably crude and woefully ineffective.

SCANDAL No. 4

Doctors of the Mind

Health and illness are essentially subjective and yet doctors insist on trying to apply an objective approach to medicine. Nowhere is this attitude more illogical and more absurd than in the field of psychiatry where doctors constantly struggle to find objective pigeon-holed categories for illnesses which are patently subjective.

In Britain today the treatment of mental illness is appalling. It is a multi-faceted scandal. But it is a scandal of horrifying proportions.

Mental illness is the biggest growth industry in Britain today. According to a recent Government White Paper there is now an unlimited demand for psychiatric help and the number of people suffering from mental illness is rising continuously and rapidly. The official figures show that between ten and fifteen per cent of the entire British population will, at some stage in their lives, suffer from mental illness severe enough to warrant their admission to a mental hospital. That means that for every eight or nine people you know there is a good chance that one of those people will need to be admitted to a mental hospital at some time.

Moreover, things are getting worse. In the last decade for which figures are available the number of patients with mental illnesses serious enough to need admission to hospital rose by over eight per cent. At any one time there are between two and three million people in Britain suffering from depression – that is approximately five per cent of the entire British population.

The figures for suicide, Britain's hidden epidemic, are frightening too. Here are some of the basic facts:

- Suicide is the third commonest cause of death in adults under the age of thirty-five – beaten only by heart disease and road accidents.

- At least one person under twenty-five commits suicide every day.
- Every year over 100,000 people try to kill themselves by taking an overdose of tablets. Would-be suicide victims now fill a hefty percentage of the emergency beds in British hospitals.
- Suicide among teenagers is increasing rapidly. It is now ten times more common for children to try to kill themselves than it was a generation ago. Every year one in every 150 girls between the ages of fifteen and nineteen will try to kill herself. The figures for young men are similar. In an average-sized school suicide is commonplace. At the rate it is going it won't be long before suicide is enemy number one for young people. In February 1987 the Samaritans claimed that there has been a twenty-four per cent increase in suicide in the last ten years.
- Attempted suicide is the commonest reason for women under thirty-five to be admitted to hospital.

With all this disturbing evidence available I don't think that any serious commentator on health matters would disagree with my claim that mental illness is the biggest health problem we have in Britain.

What makes all this particularly frightening, however, is the fact that in Britain today the treatment of patients with psychiatric problems is at best ineffective and at worst barbaric.

Twentieth-century psychiatry is more of a black art than a science and the majority of Britain's mentally ill patients would be better off if all our psychiatrists were banished to the British equivalent of Siberia. One big problem is undoubtedly the fact that although we tend to think of psychiatry as a scientific discipline psychiatry is, in truth, based more on rumour, suspicion, and gossip than on scientific evidence.

Psychiatrists are notoriously incompetent. For example, consider the way they treat the condition known as schizophrenia. This is now known to be the commonest disabling disorder to affect young adults in Britain. At least one per cent of the entire British population is schizophrenic. And yet psychiatrists can't even agree on how to define the disease let alone on a treatment. At a conference in Phoenix, USA, in 1985, which was attended by 7,000 psychiatrists from all over the world, three out of four main speakers said that schizophrenia did not exist.

In addition there is now much medico-legal evidence available to show that psychiatrists are easily conned by prisoners awaiting trial. For example, not even skilled hypnotherapists can always differentiate between patients who are in a hypnotic state and patients who are faking. In one recent experiment untrained 'patients' were able to fake paranoid schizophrenia with a seventy-two per cent success rate.

But nothing shows up the incompetence of the medical profession more than their inability to deal with the suicide epidemic that I have already outlined. Research studies have now shown quite conclusively that at least three-quarters of all the people who commit suicide consult their doctors within four weeks of killing themselves. Some of these patients consult their GPs, some consult their psychiatrists. Writing in *Modern Medicine* in February 1986 Dr Alexander L. Brown, Lecturer in the Department of General Practice at Rusholme Health Centre, Manchester, pointed out that two-thirds of the people who commit suicide will have visited their GP within a month of killing themselves while one-third will have consulted their GP within a week of their death. It is surely a terrible indictment of the quality of mental care in Britain that three-quarters of all the people who kill themselves have sought professional help. The cruellest irony, however, is the fact that many of those who kill themselves do so with pills their doctors have prescribed.

But maybe none of this is such a surprise. And maybe we shouldn't be so shocked at the inability of doctors to deal with mental problems. After all, doctors suffer more from mental illness than any other group in our society. Figures published by the Office of Population Censuses and Surveys on occupational mortality in August 1986 showed clearly that doctors commit suicide more often than any other group. Moreover, within the medical profession psychiatrists suffer more from mental illness than any other specialists, and they kill themselves more often, too.

In a sad way this seems to sum everything up. Would you trust your financial affairs to a bankrupt accountant? Would you trust your motor car to a mechanic whose own vehicle was constantly breaking down?

PSYCHOSURGERY

Psychosurgery has been performed very widely for the last half a century even though there has never been any evidence to show that it does any good. One experienced psychiatrist, who now regrets having referred patients for psychosurgery, has compared it to 'pulling the wires out of a TV set in an attempt to get a better picture'. Dr Henry Rollin, writing in the *Prison Medical Journal* in 1986 said that 'come the Day of Judgement one of the sins to which I shall have to abjectly confess is that in the early 1950s I recommended the operation [prefrontal leucotomy or lobotomy] in about twenty cases. But never again. Nothing will convince me that the operation is ever anything but unethical. I make this bold statement because I believe that to perform a destructive, irreversible operation on the brain, an organ of such infinite complexity and delicacy, is like kicking a malfunctioning computer in the hope that by doing so its efficiency will be restored.'

The type of psychosurgery or brain surgery most commonly used on psychiatric patients is prefrontal leucotomy in which a part of the brain is permanently and deliberately damaged.

The first leucotomies were performed in the 1930s when it was thought that the frontal lobes were the source of delusions in mental patients. American workers removed the frontal lobes of chimpanzees in 1935 and thought that the animals were more contented afterwards. In the following year a neurosurgeon working in Portugal tested the theory and injected alcohol into the frontal lobes of twenty schizophrenics. Since then thousands of patients have had surgical operations done to cut off their frontal lobes and the operation is still being done in Britain today. Since those who have had the operation performed are rather quiet, apparently dim and contented people few of them have complained.

The 'great' days for psychosurgery in Britain were the 1960s and the popularity of this particular brand of savagery was well described in a textbook entitled *An Introduction to Physical Methods of Treatment in Psychiatry*, written by Dr William Sargant, Physician in Charge of the Department of Psychological Medicine and Lecturer at St Thomas' Hospital Medical School, London, Dr Eliot Slater, Physician in Psychological Medicine at the National Hospital in Queen Square and Honorary Physician at the Maudsley Hospital, London, and Dr Peter Dally, Physician in Psychological Medicine at the Westminster Hospital, London. Their book has been out of print for some years.

According to these three eminent authors over 15,000 leucotomies had been performed in Britain by 1963. The operation favoured involved cutting away or simply damaging part of the brain and the operation was done for a remarkably wide range of conditions including: schizophrenia, depression, obsessional neurosis, anxiety, hysteria, eczema, asthma, chronic rheumatism, anorexia nervosa, ulcerative colitis, tuberculosis, hypertension, angina, and pain due to cancer. Leucotomies had, apparently, even been performed on patients suffering from anxiety caused by barbiturate toxicity.

The operation is described with great enthusiasm by Sargant and his two colleagues who wrote that 'it is probable that nearly every individual after the operation is happier than before'.

Despite this enthusiasm Sargant, Slater, and Dally do point out some of the drawbacks associated with the operation. They say that 'the more subtle powers of the intellect, such as its intuitive and imaginative qualities may sometimes be affected detrimentally' and the list of complications in their book includes: bedwetting, somnolence, severe and prolonged confusion, paralysis, epilepsy and changes in personality. There is also, of course, a risk that the patient will die during the operation.

Although all these dangers and problems are described in some detail it is difficult to avoid the conclusion that the authors had great regard for the value of this particular type of operation at that time (but it is to be hoped that their views have altered today). Without any real and convincing evidence based on the results of properly organized and reported clinical trials they seem happy to recommend an operation that involves the destruction of part of the brain and that carries with it enormous risks. Without proper trials it could not have been possible to be certain that any improvement noted was not simply due to the fact that the patients concerned no longer had the capacity to notice their problems. The patient who is lying stupid and senseless in bed is unlikely to complain of his eczema or his anxiety.

Sargant, Slater, and Dally wrote their book in the 1960s. Since then psychosurgery has continued to arouse considerable controversy, and criticism of this operation has been fairly widespread.

In the mid-1970s doctors suddenly seemed to wake up to the fact that no one had really done any definitive clinical trials to prove the value or danger of psychosurgery. In 1975 an editorial writer in the *Lancet*, estimating that between 200 and 300 psychosurgery operations were done each year in Britain, pointed out that many people were sceptical about the value of the neurosurgical approach to mental illness. In 1974 the World Health Organization published a book called *Protection of Human Rights in the Light of Scientific and Technological Progress in Biology and Medicine* which included the comment that 'the procedures in contemporary psychosurgery are based on inadequate or limited research and they entail many hazards. Psychosurgery has unpredictable effects on a precious organ which, even when a locus of society's discontent, should rarely need a lesion instead of special care.'

You might have thought that that would have been that and that psychosurgery would have died a natural and unmourned death. Not a bit of it. The operation lingers on and there are still surgeons around who refuse to accept that a prefrontal leucotomy is either invalid or unethical. Occasionally these surgeons produce their own scientific papers in an attempt to justify their work. Sadly, however,

95

their attempts to prove the value of their work continue to fail. Indeed, one review of 150 articles on the subject concluded that ninety per cent were of a standard below that normally required by the editors of scientific journals.

One of the most recent papers on psychosurgery to appear in a British journal was entitled simply 'Psychosurgery'. Written by Dr P. K. Bridges it appeared in an April 1984 issue of *Update*. Bridges, who works at the Geoffrey Knight Psychosurgery Unit at Brook General Hospital in London claimed in his article that 'psychosurgery is now clearly indicated in one particular therapeutic situation: that is, when there is a need for "maintenance" ECT'.

With this thought in mind I shall now turn my attention to ECT – Electroconvulsive Therapy.

ELECTROCONVULSIVE THERAPY (ECT)

When we look back a couple of hundred years we are very critical about the way that the mentally ill were treated. And our scorn is often justified. At Bethlem Royal Hospital in 1770 you could have paid a penny to watch the depressed and the manic being bled, beaten, soaked in cold water, and blasted with electricity. You could have watched noisy and troublesome patients being spun round and round on a huge wheel until they became unconscious. You would have seen patients chained together, sleeping on dirty straw. And you would have seen patients treated without either compassion or sympathy.

Today, of course, we do not deliberately beat or bleed the mentally ill. And the tranquillizing wheel has disappeared along with the dirty straw. But we do still blast the mentally ill with electricity.

It was in 1938 that the use of electricity for the treatment of mental illness was 'rediscovered'. Two Italians, called Cerletti and Bini, decided to try pumping fairly large amounts of electricity into the human brain to treat schizophrenia. They developed Electroconvulsive Therapy because they believed that epilepsy and schizophrenia could not exist together – and ECT is, of course, a sort of artificially induced epileptic attack.

In a standard Electroconvulsive Therapy session electrodes are attached to one or both sides of the patient's head and something like eighty to 100 volts are applied to the head for up to a second at a time. That amount of electricity provides a big enough current to light up a 100-watt light bulb. Not surprisingly, perhaps, in a human being it causes a brain seizure which can be traced on an electroencephalogram.

While being given the treatment patients are usually anaesthetized and given a muscle relaxant. Without the muscle relaxant contractions can be so severe that bones can be fractured or teeth chipped. An electrocardiogram is sometimes used to monitor the beating of the heart and some doctors give oxygen to reduce the risk of brain damage.

After the electric shock has been given, patients slowly regain consciousness but usually remain groggy and confused for a while. Sometimes patients complain that their ability to remember events from the past disappears. For example, Ernest Hemingway was convinced that ECT erased his personal experiences and ruined his career as a writer.

For thirty years or so psychiatrists all around the world continued to use Electroconvulsive Therapy without there ever being any evidence to show that it worked. Certainly no one ever produced any explanations showing *how* it could possibly work.

By the 1960s there was growing disquiet about this type of treatment. No one had showed that pumping electricity into the brain did any good but a number of experts had decided that it could do harm. Many patients told how they had been held down or tied down and given huge doses of electricity which had sent them into violent convulsions. It all sounded terribly barbaric – more like something from a mediaeval torture chamber than a twentieth-century hospital.

Then in 1975 the film *One Flew Over the Cuckoo's Nest* was released. In the film, based on Ken Kesey's book, actor Jack Nicholson is seen to receive electric-shock treatment. It reinforced the idea that electric-shock therapy is cruel, barbaric, and outdated. The amount of public pressure on doctors to stop giving electric shocks to psychiatric patients increased for a while. And the number of ECT treatments being given probably did fall for a few years. But then psychiatrists started to argue that they had nothing else to offer in the place of ECT. And the popularity of the technique began to rise once more.

However, even though ECT did become more 'popular' again there was still confusion and controversy about just how the treatment should be applied and for which patients it was most suitable. Numerous experiments had been done – including, it has to be said, some at Buchenwald during the Second World War – but there was still no agreement on how to get the best out of the treatment.

This confusion is best summarized in a paper entitled 'Indications for Electric-Convulsion Therapy and Its Use by Senior Psychiatrists' that was written by two psychiatrists, Gill and Lambourn, and published in the *British Medical Journal* in May 1979.

Gill and Lambourn sent a questionnaire to all senior psychiatrists in the Wessex Region of the NHS and showed that there was a considerable difference of opinion among psychiatrists about how best the treatment could be used.

First, there were great differences in the frequency with which psychiatrists used ECT. Twenty-five out of the fifty-two consultants who returned questionnaires said that they referred, on average, between one and five patients a month for ECT. Seventeen psychiatrists referred between six and ten patients and eight referred between eleven and twenty. One psychiatrist said he never used ECT and one said that he referred more than twenty patients a month.

Second, the survey also showed that there were significant differences between the reasons given for using ECT. Some said they thought it was useful in the treatment of depression, some said they used it for schizophrenia, some said they found it useful for mania.

Third, Gill and Lambourn found that more than a third of the consultants believed that temporary memory loss was invariably associated with clinically effective ECT. Despite this – and other risks associated with the treatment – less than twenty per cent of the consultants personally administered ECT.

But the most startling conclusion produced by the survey was that psychiatrists still did not agree about how to apply Electroconvulsive Therapy. Some consultants said that they preferred to give four treatments, others preferred a series of twelve treatments. Some of the consultants placed the electrodes on one side of the head. Other consultants placed the electrodes on both sides of the head. This startling survey strongly suggested that psychiatrists applying Electroconvulsive Therapy didn't have the faintest idea what they were doing.

The disquiet produced by this report led next to a major report on Electroconvulsive Therapy published by the Royal College of Psychiatrists in 1981. This report was based on 2,755 questionnaires completed by doctors using ECT.

The final blow to ECT seemed to be the conclusion in the RCP report that of the 100 NHS clinics where the researchers actually saw ECT being given none satisfied the standards that the RCP had outlined.

But it was the accusation that obsolete machinery was used which seemed to cause greatest alarm among the mandarins at the DHSS. The Secretary of State for Social Services quickly set up a working group to look into the whole question of ECT equipment. The report of this working party was published in March 1982 – just four months after the RCP study had been published.

According to this report, although over 20,000 ECT treatments were given in the United Kingdom in 1979, 'there is no agreed theoretical basis for the use of particular wave forms, frequencies, energy, rate of delivery of energy, etc.' and so 'there are no minimal performance requirements for the effective and safe use of ECT equipment to guide ECT equipment manufacturers'. In other words even in 1982 it was generally agreed that doctors did not know how ECT worked, they did not know which patients it should be given to, they did not know how it should be applied and they did not know how best to make the equipment to give the electric shocks.

The RCP produced still more shocks for the medical profession. Eighty per cent of the psychiatrists who responded said that ECT was of greatest value in the treatment of severe depression. Half thought it occasionally appropriate for schizophrenia but a quarter said that it was probably not appropriate. A quarter of the consultants who prescribed ECT had actually administered the treatment – many left the unpleasant work to junior members of their staffs who had very little training in the use of ECT.

The lack of training given to the doctors who actually administered ECT produced many problems. Very few of the doctors involved seemed to know where the electrodes should be applied and in nearly three-quarters of the clinics visited by the doctors organizing the survey the settings on the machine used to give ECT were never altered even though ECT machines are deliberately made so that the strength and pulse of the current given can be varied according to the illness and particular needs of each individual patient.

One of the most worrying aspects of the whole survey was the fact that in more than a quarter of 165 special ECT clinics visited the only machines available (and the ones being regularly used) were obsolete and did not conform to hospital safety standards. Some of the machines available had no automatic timer so that the control of the dose of electricity given depended entirely on the operator. This is potentially a very important problem because overdoses of ECT can lead to prolonged memory impairment.

With all these questions still unanswered (and, indeed, largely unasked) the Secretary of State's working party could do little. They recommended that obsolete machines be retired, that new machines be installed with safety equipment fitted and that machines should be regularly serviced (one of the more bizarre discoveries of the RCP report was that only about half the ECT equipment in regular use received any regular maintenance).

That was in 1982. Since then very little has happened.

I estimate that on average psychiatrists in Britain still refer about one new patient a week for ECT. Every year tens of thousands of patients receive a form of treatment that still hasn't been properly tested. No one has any idea why it should work, or indeed if it works. No one knows the extent of the damage it can do. No one knows when it should be given or when it should be avoided at all costs. No one knows what sort of machinery should be used or what dosage of electricity should be given. No one really knows where the electrodes should be applied.

ECT is a mystery remedy. Using ECT to treat the mentally ill is about as logical as pumping extra electricity into a malfunctioning TV set.

PSYCHOTHERAPY AND PSYCHOANALYSIS

There is a great mystique about psychotherapy but in practice psychotherapists do nothing more complicated than listen to (and occasionally talk to) their patients.

There are probably as many different psychotherapy theories as there are psychotherapists. So, for example, one psychotherapist's way of encouraging patients to learn self control is to order them to refrain from sex for a year. Another psychotherapist I know of tells bulimic patients that they have to give him money every time they vomit. The first time they have to pay a penny, then they have to double the sum on each subsequent occasion. 'Patients soon work out that it is going to cost them a fortune if they keep going – so they stop,' says the therapist who, inevitably, also charges a fee for this outrageous advice.

To become a psychotherapist you need nothing more than a little confidence, a couch, and a brass plate. Anyone, literally anyone, can set themselves up in business as a psychotherapist. You need no formal qualifications – and you certainly don't need to be a doctor. In America a pet chameleon was licensed as a psychotherapist. My cat Alice is a highly qualified psychotherapist and President of the International Association of Psychotherapy Specialists.

Given this background it is, perhaps, hardly surprising that there is no evidence available to show that psychotherapy does any good at all. One of the most comprehensive studies of psychotherapy was organized by Professor Hans Eysenck and published back in 1952. Eysenck found that two-thirds of treated neurotic patients improve within two years. But he also discovered that two-thirds of neurotics who get no treatment at all also get better within two years. Eysenck's conclusion was that expensive psychotherapy makes no difference at all to a patient's progress.

Many psychotherapists have, of course, tried to disprove Eysenck's conclusions. None has succeeded. And in 1983 psychologist Bernie Zilbergeld came to a similar conclusion. Zilbergeld, a clinical psychologist who practises in California, concluded in his book *The Shrinking of America* that the chief benefit of therapy comes from talking to a sympathetic listener. And it doesn't really matter who does the listening.

Patients, Zilbergeld pointed out, will often exaggerate the effects of psychotherapy. They do this for several reasons. They want to please the therapist. They feel grateful for feeling better. And they don't want to think that they have been wasting their money and time on a useless form of treatment.

One of the classic studies of psychotherapy which seemed to show that the treatment did work was the Cambridge Somerville Youth Study that was done in Massachusetts between 1935 and 1945. More than half of 325 problem youngsters who took part in the study said that they had benefited from psychotherapy. But when the 325 boys were followed up thirty years later by sociologist Joan McCord she found that the treated patients showed virtually no behavioural differences to a control group of 325 boys. Indeed, the boys who had been treated with psychotherapy were slightly more likely to become mentally ill, develop signs of alcoholism or commit a major crime. The control group, it should be pointed out, also consisted of boys who had in 1935 been described as 'problem youngsters'.

Even more worrying than the fact that psychotherapy just doesn't work is the fact that psychotherapists do seem to take advantage of their patients far too often. Robert Langs, Program Director of the Psychotherapy Program at Lenox Hill Hospital in New York City and the author of twenty books on psychotherapy recently concluded (referring, of course, to American patients), that 'the average consumer of therapy is likely to be influenced and perhaps overwhelmed by the emotional problems of therapists'. Langs went on to say that most patients had been 'overtly manipulated or even abused by at least one therapist'.

The continuing exploitation of patients by psychotherapists is, it seems, a continuing scandal. Most patients would probably be better off talking to a sympathetic priest or barman.

So much for psychotherapy. What about psychoanalysis? And what *is* psychoanalysis? Well, according to one leading clinician psychoanalysis is merely psychotherapy for the carriage trade. It is nothing more than an esoteric form of psychotherapy. Once again you don't need to undertake any particular training schedule in order to describe yourself as a psychoanalyst. A weekend spent reading a couple of 'pop psychology' books and a diploma bought through the post will suffice.

The classic, standard psychoanalyst follows the teachings of Sigmund Freud and claims that infantile sexual experiences play a dominant role in the development of personality disorders. He will claim that events which take place in the first few years of a patient's life are crucial to the development of his ego. Psychoanalysts are dedicated to this very rigid theory and do not accept that environmental, biochemical, genetic or electrical factors could have any influence on a patient's mental health. What psychoanalysts ignore is the fact that a large number of biographers have now discredited Freud.

It has been pointed out that there really is no sense behind Freud's argument that we are all afraid of marrying a parent and no basis for his claim that all homosexuals are liars. And a number of biographers have pointed out that Freud himself was extremely neurotic and filled with unexplained anxieties.

Those who criticize psychoanalysis in general point out that the principles of psychoanalysis are far too rigid to be of any real use to patients. Psychoanalysis is, in the words of a leading British physician, 'about as rational and scientific as scientology'. It has been said that the majority of psychoanalysts are too detached, objective, and uncaring. Practitioners have been accused of robbing patients of their self-esteem, motivation, personal sense of responsibility, and necessary illusions. 'Psychoanalysts,' says one physician, 'sometimes forgets that cigars are sometimes cigars.'

The psychoanalysts, of course, have a simple answer to all this criticism. They claim that anyone who disagrees with them has got personal problems and is denying some inner truth. They say that patients need to be broken down in order to be built up again.

Because there are relatively few psychoanalysts in Britain (most of them are in private practice where they can charge their patients enormous fees for regular sessions), psychoanalysis is probably a minor health scandal. But it is, nevertheless, a scandal for as far as I have been able to find out not one scientific paper has ever shown that psychoanalysis is of any value at all. It is impossible to write a critical analysis of a branch of medicine which does not generate any scientific literature. Listening to patients' problems undoubtedly helps them. But the listener doesn't need any special qualifications.

TRANQUILLIZERS

Just over thirty years ago – in 1954 – at the New Jersey Laboratories of Hoffman–LaRoche in America Dr Leo H. Sternbach started doing experiments with two sets of chemicals called benzophenones and heptoxdiazepines. Inspired by the commercial success of a number of existing tranquillizers Sternbach hoped that these chemicals might enable him to produce a drug with a useful pharmacological effect on the brain.

But after producing and investigating some forty new products Sternbach still hadn't managed to find anything of commercial value. Indeed, he was so disappointed by the results of his experiments that he put the final drug of the series on a shelf while he turned his attention to other more promising research projects.

Eighteen months later a laboratory spring clean resulted in this final product, known then only by its code number Ro5–0690, being sent off to Roche's Director of Pharmacological Research for proper testing.

Two months later, in July 1957, the substance had passed its first tests. It was described as being a hypnotic, a relaxant, and a sedative. And by the spring of the following year, it had been identified as an entirely new substance – a benzodiazepine.

From that point on things moved quickly. It was found that the new benzodiazepine had powerful effects as a treatment for anxiety and as an anti-convulsant. By March 1960 the preliminary tests had all been done, the American Food and Drug Administration had approved the drug and it was on the market. It was known as Librium.

That first benzodiazepine was immensely successful. Within months Roche and other companies were seeking variations on what looked like being an extremely promising theme. The new drug had been shown to relieve anxiety, to help people get to sleep and to relax tense and tight muscles. New benzodiazepines followed quickly, with Valium coming on to the market in 1963. The benzodiazepine explosion was tremendous – by 1979 there were said to be about 700 Valium-like substances available.

These new tranquillizers were greeted with enthusiasm by doctors in hospital and general practice. It seemed that the drugs were both effective and safe, and doctors who were worried about the dangers associated with the barbiturates (which were rapidly going out of fashion) were delighted to be able to prescribe these new products instead.

In the late 1960s the number of prescriptions for drugs in this group rose steadily and by 1970 the benzodiazepines and other similar drugs made up approximately 6.5 per cent of all drugs prescribed by British GPs. By 1975, when the barbiturates were the object of a campaign to reduce prescribing, the total number of prescriptions for tranquillizers was still rising – one out of every six prescriptions was for a drug in this general group.

But still the limits had not been reached. In 1977 a total of 45 million prescriptions for tranquillizers were written and almost one-fifth of all prescriptions signed by doctors were for drugs like Valium and Librium. The benzodiazepines had become the world's most popular drugs.

There were three basic reasons why the benzodiazepines proved so popular. First, most doctors in practice have grown up in a world where they are accustomed to getting their prescribing information from drug companies. As I've already explained most doctors are not trained to assess new information objectively. If a drug company tells a doctor that a drug does a particular job and is acceptably safe then the doctor will usually accept that information uncritically.

Second, by the time the benzodiazepines arrived on the scene doctors were finding it more and more difficult to hide from the fact that the barbiturates were dangerous. By the mid-1970s there was plenty of evidence to show that the barbiturates were causing an enormous addiction problem. There was an urgent need for an alternative product. And the benzodiazepines fitted the bill perfectly.

Third, doctors desperately needed the benzodiazepines. During the 1950s and 1960s the type of problem being discussed in the doctor's surgery was changing and GPs found that they were expected to deal with mental and psychological problems as well as physical problems.

The relationship between stress and disease had become common knowledge and millions of men and women had come to regard mental problems as something that could be treated. Patients who were anxious, irritable, upset, miserable and just plain unhappy all sought medical help.

Doctors had never been trained to cope with stress-induced problems. Most knew little more about anxiety and psychosomatic disease than their patients. Indeed many probably knew far less. Most doctors in practice in the 1960s and 1970s had spent as much time at medical school studying psychiatry as they had spent on tropical diseases. The benzodiazepines were an instant solution that doctors welcomed with open arms.

Amid all this enthusiasm for these new drugs a number of warning bells sounded. In 1961, just a short time after Librium was introduced into clinical practice a report appeared in *Psychopharmacologia* written by three physicians from the Veterans' Administration Hospital, Palo Alto, California. Entitled 'Withdrawal Reactions From Chlordiazepoxide [Librium]' the paper described how patients who had been taking the drug suffered from withdrawal symptoms when the drug was stopped.

That was by no means the only sign that the benzodiazepines might not be as trouble free as everyone had hoped.

In 1973 a symposium was held at the Royal Society of Medicine by a publication called the *British Clinical Journal* of which I was then the executive editor. Dr John Bonn, at the time a senior lecturer and consultant psychiatrist at St Bartholomew's and Hackney Hospitals, London, said that 'the benzodiazepines are medication to be avoided, unless the patient is under close supervision.' Dr Bonn explained that he had seen a number of benzodiazepine-dependent patients and that when these patients were weaned off their drugs they often felt much better than they had for years.

Two years later, in 1975, three doctors from the Drug Dependence Treatment Center at the Philadelphia Veterans' Administration Hospital and University of Pennsylvania, Philadelphia, published a paper in *The International Journal of the Addictions* entitled 'Misuse and Abuse of Diazepam: An Increasingly Common Medical Problem'. The three authors referred back to several papers published in the early 1970s which had documented instances of physical addiction to chlordiazepoxide and diazepam. They reported that since the end of 1972 they had noticed an increasing amount of diazepam misuse and abuse and their paper concluded: 'All physicians should know that diazepam abuse and misuse is occurring and careful attention should be given to prescribing, transporting and storing this drug.'

The addictive quality of these drugs wasn't the only problem to have surfaced, however. Back in 1968 a report published in the *Journal of the American Medical Association* dealt with eight patients who were taking diazepam in a normal daily dosage of five milligrams three or four times a day. The authors reported that seven patients had such deep depressions while on the drugs that they had developed suicidal thoughts and impulses. Two of the patients killed themselves while another two made serious attempts to commit suicide. Five of the patients showed improvements in three or four days after their diazepam had been reduced and stopped.

Then in 1972, in the *American Journal of Psychiatry* a report described how six patients on diazepam had exhibited symptoms which included apprehension, depression, insomnia, and tremulousness. Previously, the patients had all been emotionally stable and the

105

symptoms, which all started quite suddenly, were severe. When the patients were taken off diazepam their symptoms disappeared.

By the end of the 1970s the evidence damning these drugs was widely known among drug-abuse experts and, indeed, many patients. In 1979, for example, a psychiatrist testifying to a US Senate health sub-committee claimed that patients could become hooked on diazepam in as little as six weeks. The same committee also heard testimony that it is harder to kick the tranquillizer habit than it is to get off heroin. One expert witness said that tranquillizers provided America's number one drug problem, apart from alcohol.

In addition to all this evidence medical journals around the world began to carry increasing numbers of articles and reports about the problems with these drugs. Malcolm Lader, professor of psychopharmacology, reported that brain scans had produced evidence of brain damage among patients who had been taking diazepam for a number of years. Research at a neuro-psychopharmacology conference in Jerusalem in 1982 suggested that the benzodiazepines might affect the human memory. There were reports which showed that people who take benzodiazepines and then drive are particularly likely to be involved in traffic accidents. It was shown that the benzodiazepines can have an adverse effect on a patient's sex life, that they cause aggression, and that they can produce troublesome interactions if taken at the same time as tea and coffee. There was ample evidence to show that when taken by pregnant women the drugs could cause problems to the developing foetus. And in the period between 1964 and 1982 the Committee on Safety of Medicines in London received reports about well over 100 different side effects said to be related to the use of diazepam alone.

But still doctors kept on prescribing benzodiazepine tranquillizers and sleeping tablets in huge quantities. In 1985 doctors were still writing out 30 million prescriptions a year for these drugs. Every single day something like 3 million people in Britain – six per cent of the entire population – took a benzodiazepine drug. It is perhaps not surprising that the DHSS regards these figures as confidential.

During the middle and late 1970s I had written extensively about benzodiazepine tranquillizers – pointing out the dangers of addiction associated with these drugs and repeatedly explaining that every drug-abuse expert in the world seemed to agree that benzodiazepine tranquillizers are more addictive and more difficult to give up than heroin.

By the early 1980s I was getting a huge amount of mail from readers who had been taking these drugs for years and who had become addicted. In an attempt to summarize the information I had collected over ten or twelve years I wrote a book called *Life Without Tranquillizers* in which I not only described the evidence that existed, but also provided patients with advice on how best to 'kick' the tranquillizer habit.

It wasn't easy to get the book published. Several London publishers insisted that there was no tranquillizer problem in Britain. Others insisted that the tranquillizer problem was over. Eventually the book was published in 1985.

The response was extraordinary. The book went straight into the bestseller lists and I started to receive a phenomenal amount of mail from benzodiazepine addicts. In a single month I received well over 6,000 letters from tranquillizer users.

I learnt a great deal from the mail I received. I had letters from readers who had lost their homes, their families, and their jobs, and there were hundreds of letters from people who firmly believed that their health had been ruined by tranquillizers. I received letters from patients who had ended up in prison after being charged with offences that they couldn't remember committing. I had letters from readers who had struggled to give up their tranquillizers only to be told by their doctors that the benzodiazepines are perfectly safe drugs. I had letters from readers who had been told by their doctors to stop their pills suddenly – without a gradual cutting down process – and who had, as a result, suffered horrendous withdrawal symptoms. I estimated that in Britain alone there were 2.5 million people addicted to benzodiazepine.

My mail also included many letters from doctors. Some simply wrote to say that they shared my concern at the size of the problem. Others wrote to tell me of their own research work which had revealed new and additional problems associated with these drugs. For example, I had a letter from Dr Martin B. Scharf, Director of the Sleep Disorders Laboratory at Mercy Hospital in Cincinnati, Ohio. Dr Scharf was kind enough to send me a copy of a manuscript that he was about to have published in the *Journal of Clinical Psychiatry*. Over twenty pages long, the paper dealt mainly with the effect that benzodiazepine tranquillizers can have on the human memory.

Dr Scharf had found evidence to show that the benzodiazepine tranquillizers can produce anterograde amnesia – in other words patients who take drugs of this type don't just forget things that have happened to them in the past (that is retrograde amnesia) but they also forget things that happen after they have taken the drug. These findings were extremely significant.

In one experiment patients had a marked and prolonged memory loss during the day after taking a modest dose of the drug lorazepam (a commonly prescribed benzodiazepine). One patient 'lost' the whole day. In another experiment a patient who had been given a benzodiazepine had a gall-bladder attack thirty minutes after taking a tablet, but couldn't remember the attack the following morning.

In his letter to me Dr Scharf pointed out that 'the amnestic effects of the benzodiazepines no doubt represent a grossly under-reported effect. Since geriatric patients consume a disproportionately large percentage of tranquillizers and hypnotics, and considering that memory deficits in the elderly are common, a drug-induced memory impairment might go altogether unnoticed or possibly be misinterpreted as a normal consequence of ageing.'

In other words, many elderly patients had wrongly been diagnosed as senile when in fact it was the drugs they were taking which had affected their ability to think clearly.

From the thousands of letters I got during 1985 and 1986 I came to the firm conclusion that one benzodiazepine in particular, a drug called lorazepam (known to many patients by the brand name Ativan) was the most addictive and most dangerous of all the benzodiazepines. I mentioned my fears about this drug in a widely circulated medical journal and received a considerable number of letters of agreement from practising doctors all over the country.

I then sent over 100 'yellow card' reports to the Committee on Safety of Medicines, together with an extensive report detailing my fears and the evidence I had accumulated about the drug. The Committee on Safety of Medicines refused to accept the yellow cards I submitted on the grounds that I hadn't supplied enough information (even though doctors are encouraged to submit partly completed yellow cards). As I write, this drug, which I have described in *The Star* as 'the most feared drug in Britain', is still being prescribed by thousands of doctors and taken, every day, by hundreds of thousands of patients. Indeed, it is the attitude of the thousands of doctors who still prescribe lorazepam and the other benzodiazepines that puzzles and frightens me most of all.

Despite all the problems that are known to be associated with these drugs, despite the effect they have on the human memory, and despite the fact that they are more addictive than heroin, these drugs are still prescribed by the lorryload.

I estimate that in 1987 British doctors will write out between 25 million and 30 million prescriptions for these drugs.

SCANDAL No. 5

Paper Doctors

Listening to the radio recently I heard an eminent medical scientist arguing that the main problem with medicine today is that not enough money is spent on research. His claim was that if a few hundred million pounds were pumped into laboratory research then most of the problems now facing us would disappear. He implied that by spending more money we would be able to find cures for cancer, arthritis, depression, Aids, and the common cold.

He is wrong. We do not need to spend more money on medical research. If anything we need to spend less on medical research.

We need to close down our research laboratories, halt the growth of the medical-research industry and ban collecting tins for medical-research programmes. Then we need to spend our resources making sure that we take full advantage of the information that we already have available.

By spending less on research and more on practical care we would be able to improve the quality of medical care available both for our own generation and for generations to come.

Medical research is an expensive luxury that we can no longer afford.

Just consider the facts. Within the last twenty years more money has been spent on medical research than was spent in the whole of the rest of man's history on earth. And yet what have we to show for all the effort and money that has been expended? Virtually nothing.

Medicine has become full of paradoxes. The expenditure on health care has rocketed. But there has been an increase in the number of people dying in their thirties and forties. For most of us life expectancy is not increasing. Indeed, there is so much sickness around that half the adult population and a third of the child population take some form of medicament every day. We have more operating theatres than ever before. And yet there are still enormous waiting lists for essential surgery. Our surgeons are performing more and more heart operations. And yet more people than ever are dying of heart disease.

In our continuing attempts to deal with these problems we constantly increase the amount we spend on research. But it is difficult to think of any really significant advances that have been made in the last quarter of a century.

The real problem is that medical research has got completely out of hand. Most of the major breakthroughs that have been made in the last century were sheer luck. Fleming discovered penicillin by accident. Rontgen discovered X-rays by accident.

But medical research has become big business. A circus strong man would have a job to lift a *list* of all the new medical research papers published every year. The regularly published index of new research papers is inches thick and 1,000 pages long. There are so many medical journals in existence that a new scientific paper is published somewhere in the world every twenty-eight seconds. There are over 6,000 medical journals regularly being published around the world – all filled with details of new research programmes.

Because they know that they need to publish research papers if they are to have successful careers, doctors have become obsessed with research for its own sake. They have forgotten that the original purpose of research is to help patients. I spend much of my time reading and studying medical research papers. And yet I know that I can read only a fraction of one per cent of all the papers published. It has become a crazy business.

There are several specific reasons why I think we would all benefit if medical research work was stopped.

First, we need to stop and take stock of what we have already found. Believe it or not much of the research work that has been done in the last twenty years has never been analyzed. Somewhere, hidden deep in an obscure part of a medical library, there may be a new penicillin or a cure for the common cold. Or a cure for cancer. You don't have to go far to find the evidence proving that many scientific papers go unread: approximately twenty per cent of all research work is unintentionally duplicated because researchers haven't had the time to read all the published papers in their own specialized area.

Second, by putting money into collecting tins and sending money to research appeals we have encouraged thousands of our best doctors to dedicate their lives to research work. We have produced a breed of researchaholics when what we desperately need is doctors to put into practice some of the things we have already learnt.

Third, we need to redirect valuable financial resources away from expensive and unproductive research programmes and towards health-care programmes that will really save lives. In the past journalists have suggested that medical researchers are special people, fired by unusual enthusiasms and not suffering from the usual human frailties. Sadly, the truth is that as a group they are no different from any other group of professional workers. They have their own ambitions, fears, needs and weaknesses and these factors influence the direction and quality of their research. In Britain today we spend over £500 million a year on research. No one apart from the researchers would suffer if all that money was redirected elsewhere.

DISHONESTY IN RESEARCH

With enormous pressures on them to make discoveries and produce startling results a growing number of researchers are 'cooking the books' and 'fiddling the figures'.

In my book *Paper Doctors*, published in 1976, I described two examples of doctors who had been found out. The first was Dr William Summerlin, who was hired by the Sloan Ketting Institute in New York at a salary of $40,000 a year to do work on the problems of transplanting skin and overcoming rejection problems. Summerlin seemed to have made a major breakthrough in this area but no other laboratory anywhere in the world was able to duplicate his excellent results. Then, under pressure, Summerlin admitted that he had cheated. He was supposed to have transplanted skin from black mice to white mice. In fact he had simply inked in the transplant sites with a black felt-tipped pen.

The second medical trickster was Dr J. P. Sedgwick, a GP working in London's West End. Dr Sedgwick was offered £10 per card to fill in a number of trial cards showing the effects of a new hypotensive drug on the blood pressure of some of his patients. Dr Sedgwick filled in 100 cards and accepted £1,000 from the company concerned, Bayer. (See also page 34.)

Bayer became concerned when the cards were returned for not only were they still clean and unmarked but the blood-pressure figures (which all seemed to have been filled in at the same time) were identical on several sets of cards. The drug company eventually reported the doctor to the General Medical Council and in July 1975 Dr Sedgwick had the dubious distinction of being the first medical practitioner to be struck off for such unprofessional behaviour.

Since those early days of deceit, dishonesty among researchers has become sadly and regrettably all too commonplace and the journals are these days constantly reporting more and more instances of over-zealous researchers falsifying or inventing results.

In 1980, for example, the world of medicine was devastated by a series of scandals involving such prestigious centres of excellence as Yale School of Medicine, Boston's Massachusetts General Hospital and Harvard. At the Boston University Medical Center a three-year $1 million cancer research project was tainted by false data. At Cornell University Mark Spector seemed on the brink of winning a Nobel Prize for his work explaining how tumour-causing viruses could turn a cell cancerous. Then suddenly his spectacular career was in ruins. Findings that were originally described as fundamental breakthroughs were branded as fraudulent. Colleagues discovered that Spector had cunningly doctored isolated bits of cellular matter to look like things they were not.

In 1983 there was an even bigger scandal in America when Dr John Darsee who had worked as a researcher at Harvard was accused of falsifying data. Darsee had done research work on a project funded by the National Heart, Lung and Blood Institute designed to help assess the effectiveness of drugs to treat heart attacks. After the research project was discredited Harvard was asked to return the $122,371 it had received as funding.

In the autumn of 1986 Professor Michael Briggs, who had worked at an Australian University, admitted 'serious deceptions' in his research into changes in the fats in blood caused by oral contraceptives. Briggs published papers dealing with contraceptive pill side effects between 1976 and 1984 and claimed that his research work had been done at Deakin University. Two drug companies who had provided Briggs with financial backing were shocked when details of his fraudulent behaviour were revealed. Professor Briggs had, after all, been an expert adviser to the World Health Organization.

Then in November 1986 yet another fraudulent medical author was exposed. Robert Slutsky of the University of California at San Diego withdraw fifteen published papers. His action immediately put fifty-five other papers under a cloud. Towards the end of his stay at the University Slutsky had been producing new scientific papers at the rate of one every ten days.

Inevitably all this fraudulent research work leads to problems for other researchers. Once a fraudulent paper gets into the system it can be quoted hundreds of times by other researchers within months of its first publication. The *Index Medicus*, the most important listing of research papers, does not correct false information or list fraudulent authors or fraudulent papers. There is, therefore, no way for an author to check on the validity of the papers he wants to use in his own research work. In October 1986 a quick survey of papers that were known to be fraudulent revealed a total of forty-three papers published in the last five years or so. If each one of those papers was quoted by only ten other authors, then that makes 430 papers of questionable quality hiding in the world's medical literature.

Medical research is not only costly and of questionable value. Much of it, it seems, is downright misleading.

As a final footnote to this section it is also perhaps worth pointing out that in a recent analysis of research work published in his book *The Clay Pedestal* (published in the United States by Nadonna Publications) T. Preston pointed out that one survey of research work showed that almost seventy-five per cent of all the reports published contained invalid conclusions that had been based on the incorrect use of statistics.

CANCER RESEARCH

Since cancer is responsible for about twenty per cent of all the deaths in the United Kingdom it is hardly surprising that we spend an enormous amount of money on cancer research. In 1986 the Imperial Cancer Research Fund spent over £22 million on research. In the same period the Cancer Research Campaign spent about the same.

Most of this money was raised by public appeals, by collectors shaking tins in the street. Even ignoring the vast quantities of money that were spent on administration this was, I fear, largely money wasted.

For two centuries now cancer research has provided scientists with money, power, and prestige. And yet it has provided very little useful information to help us fight cancer. Since Bernard Peyrilhe did the first cancer experiment in 1773 and injected a dog with cancer fluid from a breast cancer thousands of researchers have tested new drugs and new techniques and have searched for new cures and new breakthroughs. There has certainly never been any lack of money for their efforts.

But what contribution have these researchers made to the battle against cancer? It is difficult to find any evidence that they have made any contribution at all. The number of people dying from cancer continues to rise annually. The number of different, known cancers also continues to increase.

Cancer researchers have investigated a good many possibilities and raised a good many false hopes but they have consistently failed to come up with anything useful or effective.

In contrast to all this expensive failure the epidemiologists and the

113

doctors actively treating cancer patients have come up with a host of possible answers.

Back in 1976 the World Health Organization announced that no less than eighty-five per cent of all cancers could be directly attributed to specific, known causes. They blamed cigarettes, overeating, drinking too much, too much sunlight, dangerous chemicals, and so on. In other words the preventive medicine specialists and the epidemiologists could, in 1976, tell us how to avoid seventeen out of every twenty cases of cancer.

More recently practising physicians have shown that it is possible to help cancer patients live longer and overcome their disease by adopting the right sort of mental attitude and by using the body's own healing powers.

But the epidemiologists and the practising physicians have been ignored. Their practical, straightforward, potentially effective advice has been ignored and overshadowed by the constant search for a 'magic' cure. The large cancer research organizations have misled millions into thinking that a single cure for cancer soon will be available.

I would argue that the large, well-funded, but ineffective cancer-research organizations have done a considerable amount of harm to our fight against cancer by misleading the public and by distracting public attention from the real solutions.

ANIMALS IN RESEARCH

If animals shave their whiskers then their brains don't develop properly.

Isn't that interesting? I bet you're glad I told you that. I know this fascinating fact because a team of research scientists working at the University of Pittsburg School of Medicine has just completed a research project designed to find out what happens when rats' whiskers are shaved. During the experiment a technician shaved the rats' whiskers every day with a pair of tiny scissors. And the researchers then found that the rats' brains didn't develop properly.

When I was researching my book *Paper Doctors*, about a dozen years ago, I was horrified by the number of medical researchers who spend their time and our money on research projects which have no practical value. There was the Cambridge psychologist who deliberately blinded a monkey and studied her behaviour for six years. There were the researchers who kept their animals in terribly cramped and inadequate conditions. And there were the researchers who maimed and destroyed hundreds of animals simply so that they could test new cosmetics. Some researchers deprived animals of food and water. Others subjected their defenceless victims to terrible pain. Many of the experiments were done by students who could have just as easily learned from filmed experiments or from well-illustrated textbooks.

At the time I was by no means the only writer to be disgusted by what was going on in the name of scientific research. Many other authors also aroused public opinion by describing cruel, vicious and entirely unnecessary experiments. Politicians got involved. Newspapers carried huge feature articles on the subject of vivisection. And there were demonstrations and marches outside many laboratories.

As a result of all this publicity and of the promises that were made I assumed that researchers would stop using so many animals in their experiments. Naively I took it for granted that the Home Office would clamp down on the number of licences given to researchers. But while researching this book I was horrified to learn that every year British scientists still conduct an enormous number of entirely unnecessary experiments. The latest figures show that there are still well over 4 million animal experiments conducted every year in Britain. Most of those experiments are performed on cats, dogs, rabbits, guinea pigs, mice, rats, hamsters, and monkeys. Many of those animals are kept in terrible conditions. Hundreds of thousands are subjected to dreadful pain and fearful suffering. (For example, in February 1985 the Royal College of Surgeons of England was found guilty and fined £250 for causing unnecessary suffering to a laboratory monkey. The court was told that monkeys used in experiments were kept in three-foot square aluminium cages. Because of an inadequate heating system the temperature inside the cages had soared from 85°F to 92°F.) The lucky ones are the ones which are killed during the early stages of an experiment.

Despite all the publicity and controversy, despite the public outcry in the past, despite the accusations of scandal, there are still nearly as many animal experiments conducted today as there were ten years ago.

The researchers who conduct these experiments usually argue that their work will benefit mankind. They dismiss protestors as ignorant and unreasonable. They claim that it is necessary to maim, torture, and kill animals in order to push back the frontiers of medical science.

To try and assess the value of these claims I took a long, hard look at exactly what medical-research workers are doing with animals these days. I was not impressed by what I found.

In the *Journal of the Royal Society of Medicine*, for example, I found the following three papers:

115

a) 'Effects of Vibration, Noise and Restraint on Heart Rate, Blood Pressure, and Renal Blood Flow in the Pig.'

It is difficult to see the point in this particular experiment. If you happen to be a pig and you happen to operate a road drill then this sort of research work is probably useful to you. Otherwise I fail to see its significance.

b) 'Exercise in Non-mammalian Vertebrates: A Review.'

In case you, like me, are not too sure of the purpose of this research, I'll quote the final sentence of the author's conclusions: 'Because of their oxygen-conserving response that can be brought into operation when under water, tufted ducks can vary heart rate by a factor of twenty or more, depending on whether they are flying or whether they are trapped under water.'

Now, does it make sense?

c) 'Effect of Experimental Hypothyroidism on Hearing in Adult Guinea Pigs.'

I suppose this paper might be of great significance if you happen to be a guinea pig with a thyroid problem.

Those three papers seem more comical than threatening. So let me continue with an account of the work of one of Britain's most respected scientists, Professor Colin Blakemore.

Blakemore leads a research team at Oxford University and for some time his work has been sponsored by the Medical Research Council. For the best part of the last twenty years he has been conducting research into vision.

For example, in 1986 Blakemore and a colleague published a paper entitled 'Organization of the Visual Pathways in the New-born Kitten'.

These two intrepid researchers used thirteen new-born kittens in their experiment. Each kitten was injected with chemicals. Some of the kittens had the chemicals injected directly into the part of their brain that helps to provide sight. Twenty-four hours later the kittens were killed. And their brains dissected.

Blakemore and his colleague concluded that they 'had gained further information about the organization of the visual pathways in the new-born kitten before the onset of visual activity'. At the end of the paper the two scientists listed no less than eighty-eight presumably relevant references – most of them dealing with similar experiments with cats and kittens. This experiment was similar to many conducted by Blakemore and his colleagues.

For example, in 1985, David Price, who works with Blakemore, reported on an experiment in which a total of seventeen kittens were used. Five of the kittens were reared in complete darkness from the day they were born. As far as I can see the conclusion Price came to at the end of his research was that kittens do not develop normally when they are reared in the dark.

In 1985 the *Journal of Neuroscience* published a paper by Blakemore and Price entitled 'The Postnatal Development of the Association Projection from Visual Cortical Area Seventeen to Area Eighteen in the Cat'. As usual the experiment was funded by the Medical Research Council.

In this experiment eighteen domestic tabby kittens were used at various ages. Two of them were binocularly deprived by suturing the conjunctivae and eyelids. For 'binocularly deprived' you can substitute 'blinded'. Albeit temporarily. Their eyes were sewn up.

Also in 1985 Blakemore and two colleagues published an article in the *Journal of Comparative Neurology*. For this research project they used fifty-nine golden hamsters. In about half the animals the left eye was removed on the day of birth. (The authors seem to me to be rather sloppy scientists – they actually say 'about half'.) The eyes which remained were injected with chemicals.

And so it goes on. I have a huge file of papers by Blakemore and his colleagues. They sew up the eyelids of animals. They inject brains. And to what end? I don't know. I have read many of Blakemore's papers and I cannot think of any excuse for what this man does in the name of science. Indeed, Blakemore claims that his work does not have to be justified in clinical terms. The Medical Research Council funds Blakemore's terrible experiments, but I challenge either the MRC or Blakemore himself to point to a single human being or animal and say that that person has benefited because of his work.

Personally I despise such scientists. I do not believe that this work has any clinical value. Human beings have little in common with animals and the results of experiments such as these cannot easily be applied to human beings. Even if I were prepared to accept that such experiments helped further medicine, I would find the experiments difficult to accept. I do not believe that such experiments have made any valid contribution and I am appalled that the Medical Research Council should support such work.

Finally, as evidence to support my claim that animal research is irrelevant to human beings, I will just mention a story which illustrates only too vividly the uselessness of animal research work.

In 1959 a Scots doctor told the drug company E. R. Squibb and Sons that a drug that they had prepared for the treatment of diarrhoea damaged the eyesight of rabbits. Squibb's own scientists then subsequently found that the drug blinded and killed two calves. In 1963 they found that the drug blinded and killed grown cattle. Also in 1963 they found that the drug killed or paralyzed dogs. Nevertheless that same year Squibb launched the drug on the market and in 1965 they obtained approval to sell the drug for use in humans.

When in the early 1980s Squibb was taken to court by a woman who lost her sight and became paralyzed after taking the drug the drug company denied negligence saying that they knew of no evidence that the drug had adverse effects on human beings.

They apparently dismissed the animal research as irrelevant since animals are different to humans. I rest my case. All animal research is an affront to human dignity – let alone the animals'.

PATIENTS IN RESEARCH

When an eighty-four-year-old woman called Margaret Wigley died in a large hospital in Birmingham, after unknowingly taking part in a drug trial, many patients were startled that such a thing could happen in Britain in the 1980s. Most probably they thought that Mengele was the only doctor ever to have used patients for experiments without first obtaining their consent. But Mengele was just one among many thousands of doctors who have, over the years, used and abused their patients. Hundreds of far more eminent physicians and surgeons have done awful things to their patients.

What about the psychologist at Johns Hopkins University who did experiments with new-born babies? His work involved dropping new-born children just as they were falling asleep.

Or what about the psychologist who encouraged a small boy to befriend a pet rat and then made a loud noise every time the boy moved to pick up the rat. Soon the small boy, called Albert, began to cry whenever his pet rat appeared. Eventually the boy became so disturbed that he was frightened by just about anything and everything. The researcher was devastated when the small boy was adopted and taken away from his laboratory.

Or what about the experiments conducted by Dr Myrtle B. McGraw of Columbia University in America? McGraw used a total of forty-two babies aged between eleven days and two and a half years in her experiments reported in the *Journal of Paediatrics*. What did McGraw do with these unfortunate babies? She held them under water to see how they responded.

In her article she reported that 'the movements of the extremities are of the struggling order' and went on to say that the babies 'clutch at the experimenter's hand'. She also noticed, apparently with some surprise, that the babies tried to wipe the water from their faces. And she seemed positively amazed that 'the ingestion of fluid was considerable and the infant would cough or otherwise show respiratory disturbance'.

In Italy doctors have put drops into the eyes of women in order to study the formation of experimental cataracts. A professor in Milan gave children drugs to stop them making a natural recovery from viral hepatitis.

Spend an hour or two flicking through the world's medical journals and it is possible to find scores of experiments as foul and offensive as these. Over the years some of the world's leading researchers have taken part in experiments that would have made even Mengele blush with shame.

But until the death of Margaret Wigley in that hospital in Birmingham became widely known most observers probably thought that clinical trials endangering patients were rare in Britain in the 1980s.

Sadly, the truth is that experiments involving unwitting patients are commonplace in Britain.

Most such experiments are conducted in considerable secrecy, of course, and even when the results are published it is sometimes difficult to tell whether or not patients were invited to give their consent. But sometimes even when patients do give their consent there are genuine reasons for concern.

Take, for example, the case of Dr Richard Woodland. In 1984 the medical newspaper *Pulse* reported that Dr Woodland had for years used Electroconvulsive Therapy on his patients in general practice. According to the report he had given more than 10,000 treatments to his patients in Paignton, Devon, and then in London. At one time about one in seven of the patients on Dr Woodland's list were receiving treatment with ECT.

Dr Woodland used this controversial treatment for a number of problems and claimed it helped patients suffering from arthritis, indigestion, irritable bowel syndrome, and aphthous ulcers. He has admitted that he didn't always obtain informed consent from his patients but even when he did tell his patients what he was planning to do and when they did understand his plans, can his actions be justified?

Many other doctors think not. Dr Woodland has addressed meetings of doctors where the audiences have walked out on him. He has described his work as 'research' and has said that stricter controls on research would limit basic freedoms to practise medicine.

But what about the rights of patients? Like many other physicians Dr Woodland seems to me to put those rights fairly low down on his list of personal priorities.

Dr Woodland may be a slightly unusual doctor, but there are thousands of doctors practising in Britain today who regularly use their patients in experiments involving new drug therapies. In general practice, in particular, there are virtually no rules stopping doctors from using their patients for new drug trials. And since drug companies sometimes pay doctors quite generously for this work it is perhaps hardly surprising that so many doctors fall to temptation. Many of the patients who suffer unpleasant or serious side effects are never even aware that they have taken part in an experiment. GPs often fail to tell their patients when they are trying an entirely new drug. When the patient is asked to take part in a trial the chances are that his full, knowing consent will not be obtained. Too often patients agree to take part in experiments because they do not understand that there are safe and effective alternatives available; they do not understand that the doctor inviting them to be guinea pigs is using them for his own personal profit.

And the risks involved during drug trials can be considerable. In February 1987 the *British Medical Journal* published a paper which described how, when three doctors at the University of Manchester conducted a trial for a drug company three out of twelve paid volunteers became ill. That sort of level of risk is, in my view, by no means unusual.

In the past some medical research was undoubtedly essential. Without experiments no new products would have ever been marketed and no new treatments would have ever been devised. But I firmly believe that the only really acceptable experiments are the ones which involve patients who are genuinely ill, and for whom no available, suitable, useful treatment can be found. Under those special circumstances, if the patient agrees to try out a new drug, then the risks are acceptable. The patient can benefit from the experiment.

In the majority of experiments, however, a new product or a new treatment is tried for personal or commercial reasons. There are usually other, accepted treatments available but the doctor or drug company involved wants to do research that will help in the production of scientific papers and, maybe, help bring a new and potentially profitable product on to the market.

In the *Journal of the American Medical Association* in March 1986 there appeared an article entitled 'Mammon and Medicine: the Rewards of Clinical Trials'. The article was written by Dr Howard M. Spiro. At the start of his article Dr Spiro confessed: 'I could get most of my patients to participate in almost any kind of clinical study. They would swallow new drugs, receive infusions of calcium or glucagon, or even embrace oesophageal or rectal catheters because they had faith in my goodwill or, I now fear, because they wanted to please me.' Dr Spiro has seen the light. He now believes that patients should be told *why* they are being invited to take part in clinical trials. Sadly, many thousands of British doctors do not yet agree with him.

SCANDAL No. 6

THE NHS – The Land of Waste

Doctors, nurses, administrators, and organizations representing patients are constantly clamouring for more money to be pumped into the National Health Service. Every time a hospital ward has to close or a patient doesn't get treated well there are choirs of angry voices screaming for the government to spend more on health care. It doesn't matter what government is in power, the arguments are always the same.

But the truth is that the NHS doesn't need any more money in order to provide the sort of service we would all like. It has plenty of money already. But much of it is wasted.

We have a rotten and crumbling health service not because there isn't enough money being poured into it, but because the money that is made available is not used wisely.

Through a mixture of incompetence and dishonesty the NHS wastes several billion pounds every year. If that money wasn't wasted, it could be used to cut waiting lists, open better hospitals, provide more district nurses, and generally provide the sort of service that most of us would like to see.

Health care is getting more and more expensive.

In 1948 we spent 4.2 per cent of our entire Gross National Product on the National Health Service. We now spend six per cent of our Gross National Product on the NHS. In cash terms that means £20,000 million a year. It's an enormous amount of money. And yet the people who spend it on our behalf do not spend it wisely.

Doctors and administrators who, in their private lives, have to watch the pennies and the pounds, find themselves handling tens of millions of pounds and brushing aside as irrelevant, unnecessary, and inconsequential suggestions for saving the odd million or two.

Few of those working in the NHS know anything at all about cost-effectiveness or efficiency. A recent survey showed that only a third of hospital consultants know that every single outpatient

122

attendance costs at least £19. Only eleven per cent of GPs know that it costs £85 a day (minimum!) just to keep a patient in hospital. Only a fifth of all GPs know that the average cost of an item prescribed by a general practitioner is £4. (These figures are taken from an editorial which appeared in the journal *Update* in November 1986. A more complete analysis of the survey appeared in the journal *Medical Education* in 1985.)

When attempts are made to cut down on the waste in the NHS, doctors, nurses, and patients often protest as though the cuts were designed to reduce the effectiveness of clinical services. For example, the *Daily Telegraph* recently included on its letters' page a communication from Jack Magell, a consultant surgeon in Blackburn, Lancashire. 'In recent months,' wrote Mr Magell indignantly, 'senior doctors in the hospital service have been encouraged to undertake budgetary control of their units. It would appear that as a finite amount of money will be available, they will somehow have to manage within this budget. It seems to me that it is not a doctor's job to ration resources. I would refuse to tell a patient that his treatment could not proceed because the money had run out.'

This sort of attitude is by no means uncommon. And inevitably it means that genuine attempts to save money so that improvements in the health service can be made meet with obstruction rather than enthusiasm. Doctors assume that because they work in medicine they are entitled to work without any form of budgetary control at all. They regard words such as 'efficiency' with undisguised distaste. They are often far more liberal with the nation's resources than they ever would be with their own. I wonder if Mr Magell would object if his family constantly left fires and lights burning and regularly threw out items of household equipment with the rubbish? Or would he regard simple household management as offensive and intrusive?

This conceit, this living in cloud-cuckoo-land, this unwillingness to accept that health care must obey the same general economic rules as other aspects of life, does not just affect doctors. It affects nurses, technicians, and administrators. Together their lack of interest in financial controls means that the NHS leviathan now loses countless millions of pounds every day.

Decisions about the day-to-day use of resources are made without any real thought being given to cost-effectiveness. There is so much money involved in running the NHS, and so much of it is regularly wasted, that those who practise within its comforting arms feel content to carry on without thinking about the financial consequences of their activities. And yet, so often, it is easy to see how money could be saved. Take, for example, the relatively minor and apparently insignificant task of recruitment advertising.

In March 1985 the Secretary of State for Social Services, Norman Fowler, felt it necessary to issue guidance to health authorities to tell them how best to recruit new staff without wasting unnecessary money.

He suggested that health authorities should not advertise posts in more than one journal (unless there was a statutory requirement to do so), should only include necessary information in advertisements, should use advertising agencies which would give a discount on advertising rates, should consider using Job Centres for local recruitment and should not use display advertising unnecessarily. By following those simple and perfectly reasonable guidelines Mr Fowler estimated that the NHS would save £4 million a year.

I find it difficult to understand why the highly paid administrators responsible for placing recruitment advertising should need a circular from the Secretary of State to encourage them to obey such obvious and commonsensical guidelines.

On the pages which follow I have detailed a few of the other ways in which NHS money is regularly wasted.

A SURFEIT OF ADMINISTRATORS

Right at the top of the administrative hierarchy of today's NHS there is a Secretary of State for Social Services – an elected politician who may or may not know anything at all about health care. For the period of his or her appointment the Secretary of State is in total charge of the Personal Social Services, the Social Security Services, and the NHS.

The Secretary of State is assisted in administrative duties by the Department of Health and Social Security, which itself comprises a large chunk of the civil service and which is mainly centred in offices at the Elephant and Castle in London. The DHSS was formed in 1968 by a shotgun marriage which united the Ministry of Health and the Ministry of Social Security. The Secretary of State was originally known as the Secretary of State for Health and Social Services but somewhere along the line a year or two ago the word 'Health' was, perhaps significantly, dropped from the title. The DHSS does not itself provide or administer any practical health services but exists solely to ensure that other administrative groups provide such services.

The number of full-time highly paid administrators employed in the DHSS's central offices is naturally large. Understanding precisely what each member of the élite bureaucracy does is next to impossible for a mere medical observer. For example, in one of its own explanatory publications the DHSS points out that the Chief Medical Adviser to Social Security Services has the status of a Deputy Chief Medical Officer in the DHSS and the Deputy Chief Medical Adviser that of Senior Principal Medical Officer.

For all practical purposes the administrators employed at the DHSS's central office are beyond criticism and when a Commons Select Committee dared to point out that the DHSS's long-term strategic planning and monitoring of health and social services was 'ineffective and nonexistent', the DHSS immediately responded with a pungent attack on the committee, pointing out that 'since they did not ask for information about the Department's machinery for strategic policy-making they were not told about it'. Other observers (myself included) have asked about this machinery but have still failed to obtain any useful information.

With the aid of the DHSS the Secretary of State is, as I have already explained, responsible for three distinct types of service.

The Social Security section is the branch of the tree responsible for handing out pensions, sickness benefits, and so on and in an average year in the late 1980s it will get through about £20,000 million: a massive sum that would work out at about £400 for every man, woman and child in the country if the administration did not use up a substantial part of the total.

Personal Social Services, which form the second branch, are handled by local authorities and consist of the provision of old people's homes, social workers, home helps, and other non-medical aids. The third branch of the DHSS is the NHS – the branch with which this book is concerned.

The highest tier in the NHS administration which has any practical responsibility and any real contact with sick people consists of the fourteen Regional Health Authorities which are responsible for long-term planning in their own regions. They do have some responsibility for providing specialist facilities (such as blood-transfusion services) and they have the authority to appoint consultants in all specialities but their main task is to supervise the provision of health-care services within their region.

Each Regional Health Authority has, in addition to a paid chairman, a team of administrative officers which runs the RHA on behalf of the committee members. Each RHA also has a wide range of advisory groups and committees of health professionals. There are quite a number of these committees – and all are expensive to run. One RHA was so dismayed when it discovered that its Medical Advisory Committee had itself got thirty-nine sub-committees that it set up another special sub-committee to look into the number of committees in existence. It now has forty sub-committees.

Beneath the RHAs in the hierarchy there are about 200 District Health Authorities which are responsible for the day-to-day management of local hospitals, health clinics, nursing services, and school health services. Each District Health Authority is, of course, well equipped with huge teams of administrators, advisors, and committees.

For years now this cumbersome and inefficient organization has grown steadily larger and larger. From time to time it has arranged reorganizations which have changed nothing and ordered reviews which have been ignored. Within this system there are impenetrable layers of administration. It is like something that Huxley, Orwell or Kafka might have created. There are countless thousands of individuals with authority but none with responsibility. Reports and documents circulate within the many departments and sub-departments in an endless and fruitless whirl of apparent activity. None of it has anything to do with health, medicine, sickness or people. It is all incredibly cumbersome, top heavy, and unnecessary and many well-qualified outside experts have been astonished at the way it has been allowed to grow unhindered.

In 1975 there were 35,460 doctors working in NHS hospitals. By 1985 there were 43,495 doctors. A rise of twenty-three per cent.

In 1975 there were 335,753 nurses working in NHS hospitals. By 1985 there were 352,532 nurses working in NHS hospitals. A rise of five per cent.

In 1975 there were, on average, 387,632 beds available in NHS hospitals. By 1985 the number of available beds had fallen to 325,487 – a drop of sixteen per cent.

In 1975 there were 588,483 patients on in-patient waiting lists. By 1985 there were 680,244 patients on in-patient waiting lists. A rise of sixteen per cent.

But in that same ten-year period the number of administrators in NHS hospitals (and this does not count the administrators working at the DHSS headquarters, or the administrators working at RHA headquarters or the number of administrators working at DHA headquarters) had risen from 17,215 to 24,115. That is a massive forty per cent rise!

The NHS is now the largest employer in Europe. It has well over a million employees. It is expanding rapidly. Most of the expansion is in administrative staff. In the summer of 1987 Dr Max Gammon, a GP in South London, produced a report for the St Michael's Organization. His report showed that although the number of nurses working in the NHS had increased between 1974 and 1984 instead of benefiting patients the extra manpower had been taken up in performing administrative work. And all the time the number of patients being treated by the NHS is falling and the number of people waiting for treatment is rising. Inevitably, when cuts are made it is never administrators who are made redundant.

The evidence suggests to me that the DHSS, the Regional Health Authorities and the District Health Authorities are all failing to do their work properly. If these massive layers of administration worked efficiently then the NHS would be far more efficient.

Having carefully studied the workings of the NHS for over two decades, I am convinced that the whole structure would benefit if ninety-nine per cent of the people employed by the DHSS, the Regional Health Authorities and the District Health Authorities were found other, more constructive work. There must be thousands of public lavatories in Britain which need cleaning.

I would recommend firing all regional and district administrators and keeping a skeleton staff of perhaps 200 minor administrators in London. No patients would suffer and the release of extra money for essential patient care would mean that millions of patients would benefit instantly. The overall management of NHS hospitals and clinics could easily be organized at local level with some guidance from the skeleton crew at the DHSS offices. The allocation of financial resources could be managed by a small, expert financial team at the Treasury. The provision of new facilities could be orchestrated by local politicians and professionals.

The DHSS, as we know it today, serves no useful purpose. It simply exists and acts as a massive drain on NHS resources.

UNNECESSARY TESTS AND INVESTIGATIONS

Every year doctors waste millions and millions of pounds by ordering unnecessary tests and investigations.

In July 1979 the *British Medical Journal* published an article entitled 'Costs of Unnecessary Tests'. The article was written by Dr Gerald Sandler, a consultant physician at Barnsley District General Hospital.

During a two-year period Dr Sandler kept a careful check on 630 patients seen in outpatient departments at one hospital. He found that the most important factor in preparing a diagnosis and arranging treatment was the information given to the doctor by the patient. This basic oral exchange of information decided fifty-six per cent of all diagnoses and forty-six per cent of all treatment. In nearly one half of the 630 patients no extra tests and investigations were needed.

Physical examinations were responsible for another big chunk of the diagnoses made and the management programmes ordered. Laboratory tests and investigations contributed to less than one per cent of all the diagnoses made.

Dr Sandler concluded that the annual cost of the useless investigations ordered on his 630 patients was a massive £3,598.72.

'In the Barnsley District General Hospital,' wrote Dr Sandler, 'an annual saving of £2,822 could have been achieved in one medical clinic by omitting routine investigations in patients in whom the diagnosis had already been made on the basis of the history and clinical examination. The justification for any investigation should surely be to answer a specific clinical question relating to diagnosis and management only when there is doubt as to either, or to measure the effect of treatment that cannot be assessed on symptoms or signs alone. Where these requirements are not operative, however, and where the result of the investigation, whether positive or negative, is unlikely to change either the diagnosis or management of the patient, there can be little justification for asking for it.'

Sadly, Dr Sandler probably wasted his time writing his article. Nothing was changed as a result.

In April 1987 the *British Medical Journal* published an article entitled 'Can More Efficient Use Be Made of X-Ray Examinations in the Accident and Emergency Department?' This article was written by three doctors from the Accident and Emergency Department at Walton Hospital in Liverpool. These three doctors concluded that new guidelines they had introduced, explaining when X-rays should be ordered at their hospital, had saved £18,000 a year without diminishing the quality of care provided.

So, in Barnsley a doctor has been saving money on his outpatient tests and investigations for about nine years and in Liverpool savings in the X-ray department at one hospital have been accumulating for one year.

But what has been happening at other hospitals in Britain? Probably nothing. The available evidence all suggests that doctors are not interested in saving money by cutting out useless and unnecessary tests (even when those unnecessary tests may put patients at risk – see page 73). Indeed, most doctors do not even know how much tests and investigations cost – let alone how much could be saved by cutting out unnecessary tests and investigations.

In an article published in the journal *Medical Education* in 1985 and entitled 'Doctors' Knowledge of the Cost of Medical Care' Dr Fowkes showed just how ignorant doctors are.

Fowkes gave an anonymous multiple-choice questionnaire to hospital clinicians who were attending a ward round in a teaching hospital, to GPs attending a conference on medical auditing and medical students attending a lecture. There were twenty questions concerned with the costs of everyday procedures.

Only sixteen per cent of hospital clinicians and eleven per cent of GPs had any real idea of the cost of a simple, straightforward, commonly performed thyroid test. But then is this ignorance all that surprising? For not even the DHSS itself can give precise figures for the costs of tests and investigations. The figures vary enormously from hospital to hospital and from laboratory to laboratory. A barium-meal X-ray examination, for example, can cost anything from £20 to £30. And pregnancy tests can cost between around £5 and around £10. Or maybe £12. Or maybe more. No one seems to know. Is it, perhaps, any wonder that most doctors just don't care and order tests and investigations as if their cost was totally irrelevant?

It is, believe it or not, still quite normal in many hospitals for doctors in a casualty department to order a set of tests when a patient is admitted through their department and for a ward doctor to then order exactly the same set of tests again when the patient is moved on to the ward.

You will probably not be surprised to hear that it is also standard practice for doctors to order a completely new set of routine tests if a patient arrives at their hospital from another hospital. If you have a chest X-ray and full blood count done at hospital A on Tuesday and then travel to hospital B with your X-rays and blood results, the doctors at hospital B will insist on repeating all the tests that you've already been through. This isn't unusual or odd. Although there is no logical reason for it, it is widely accepted as standard practice within the NHS.

DRUGS

We currently spend around £1,500 million a year on drugs. Approximately one half of that money is wasted.

Doctors overprescribe, they give patients repeat prescriptions that they don't need, they prescribe drugs that are unnecessary and they prescribe drugs that are useless. In a previous part of this book (see page 56) I described some of the ways in which doctors waste money by prescribing carelessly or through ignorance.

But doctors don't just waste money by prescribing too many drugs and by prescribing drugs that don't work. They also waste money by prescribing expensive brand-name versions of drugs that are readily available in other, cheaper forms. The Government's limited list of cheap drugs – below – involves only a small number of drugs and has little overall effect.

In 1975 when I wrote my first book *The Medicine Men* I pointed out that huge quantities of NHS money are wasted on brand-name drugs. At that time, for example, prednisolone from the cheapest source cost less than 30 pence for 100 five-milligram tablets, while manufacturers were charging up to 94 pence for the same number of branded tablets. Other drugs with a similar effectiveness in the treatment of conditions such as rheumatoid arthritis cost £5.14 per hundred tablets.

Aware of the danger to their profits should doctors stop prescribing brand-name versions and start prescribing drugs by the generic or chemical names, throughout the 1970s and early 1980s drug companies ran a vigorous campaign to persuade doctors that generic drugs were neither as safe nor as effective as branded products.

For example, the *British Medical Journal* carried an advertisement for an oral hypoglycaemic (a product used in the treatment and control of diabetes) which included a picture of two sugar cubes and a dice and the advertising line: 'It's a gamble treating diabetes with so called "equivalents" of Diabinese, the original chlorpropamide.'

The drug-company advertising worked well and even though there was fairly widespread agreement among drug experts that branded products offered no advantage over non-branded products, doctors continued to prefer to prescribe the more expensive versions.

Throughout the early 1980s doctors continued to overprescribe and to prescribe expensive, inessential drugs in a scandalously carefree manner. It became commonplace for hoards of unused drugs to be found in the bathrooms of elderly patients. The cost of the average prescription rose steadily at a rate that far exceeded the average increase in the cost of living. Doctors were prescription-happy and the NHS was being bled to death by their profligate penpushing.

Eventually, in 1985, the Government decided that it had had enough. Attempts to persuade doctors to cut down their prescribing had fallen on deaf ears. To the amazement of the medical profession and the drugs industry (both of which have extraordinarily powerful lobby groups) the Secretary of State for Social Services, Norman Fowler, announced that he planned to cut back the number of drugs that doctors could prescribe.

Explaining that the cuts would save millions of pounds of NHS money Fowler announced that he intended to cut back on the number of antacids, cough medicines, laxatives, and tranquillizers available to doctors. All the drugs involved were members of groups

130

that have repeatedly been described by authoritative, independent experts as useless or unnecessary or potentially harmful.

The response from the drugs industry and the medical profession was dramatic. Doctors immediately threw up their arms in horror and complained that their patients would suffer and probably die. Many talked emotionally about 'the freedom to prescribe' and about the problems that would be facing the poor and the elderly. It was talked about as though it were the end of the NHS.

The powerful drugs industry immediately started a campaign designed to get the Government to change its mind. They were not, of course, concerned about their own profits. They were concerned for the hardship patients would face.

The joint campaign by Britain's doctors (led inevitably by the all-powerful British Medical Association) and the drugs industry led to a weakening of the proposals. The Government reduced the number of drugs destined for the new 'black list'.

The truth was, of course, that the proposed cuts never threatened a single patient. Two years later no doctor could point to a single patient whose life had been endangered or threatened by the cuts. And yet tens of millions of pounds had been saved.

The drugs industry had been up in arms about the cuts because they knew that they were about to lose some of their best-selling lines. For years drug companies had enjoyed the freedom to produce a seemingly endless stream of useless and unnecessary drugs. They had ruthlessly encouraged doctors to waste huge sums of money on prescribing expensive versions of drugs that no one needed.

When the restrictions were introduced in Britain in 1985, there were thousands of drugs available for doctors to prescribe and yet the World Health Organization's list of essential drugs ran to only 200 products. Doctors had for years enjoyed the right to prescribe anything they liked. The new legislation merely curtailed that freedom a little, forcing doctors to prescribe cheaper versions of available drugs.

Now that the restrictions have been shown to have worked – and not to have had any adverse effects on patients – it is to be hoped that the Government will press on and put many more drugs on the 'black list'.

Doctors have shown that as a profession they are more closely linked to the drugs industry than to the needs and interests of their patients; they have shown an inability to prescribe sensibly or rationally.

Despite the Government's 1985 initiative there is still a long way to go. If doctors were forced to prescribe more logically, then the NHS would save at least £750 million a year and patients in Britain would be far, far healthier than they are at present. Anyone who doubts my assertion that doctors do not understand the cost of the drugs they prescribe should study a survey by Rowe and MacVicar which appeared in the *Journal of Clinical and Hospital Pharmacy* in 1986. Rowe and MacVicar asked thirty trainee GPs and twenty hospital doctors to estimate the cost of a month's supply for some drugs and a week's course of some antibiotics. The drugs were all common ones and the authors defined an 'accurate' assessment of cost as anything between half and twice the true cost. Only seventeen out of fifty doctors got the price of indomethacin right (the true cost was at the time 100p for three 25 milligram capsules for a month – doctors' estimates varied between 70p and 500p). Two per cent of the doctors got the price right for diazepam and nitrazepam. Twenty-six per cent of the doctors got the price right (remember they were allowed a wide range) for tetracycline. And none of the doctors got the price right for the diuretics bendrofluazide and frusemide.

FIDDLES AND THEFT

At a conference on security in the NHS, organized by the National Association of Health Authorities in 1983, the then Junior Health Minister Mr Geoffrey Finsberg was told that the NHS is losing millions of pounds to thieves.

Mr Ernest Parkinson, Chairman and Chief Executive of the National Association of Health Service Security Officers, pointed out that anything between ten and twenty per cent of the value of linen in circulation in NHS hospitals is lost every year. Theft, he said, is mostly to blame. Baby clothes and tea towels disappear particularly rapidly.

Mr Finsberg pointed out that if the losses could be cut by five per cent then that would release enough money to employ another 600 nurses or another 200 doctors.

But Mr Parkinson wasn't solely concerned with linen. He also said that he believed that at least £3.6 millions' worth of food is stolen every year and he had some specific and fairly startling examples of dishonesty:

- In one hospital thirty washing machines cost £20,000 to service during one twelve-month period. That £20,000 could have bought two new machines for each one serviced.
- In another hospital eleven painters used 2,985 five-litre cans of paint while in another hospital eight painters, who worked more hours, used 270 five-litre cans of paint.

132

By 1984 concern about the thefts in NHS hospitals was rising even more rapidly. Mr Neil Whalley, Assistant Treasurer for Halton Health Authority, showed that savings of at least ten and often twenty-five per cent or more could be saved in NHS transport alone simply by cutting out dishonest or incompetent practices. That would mean an overall saving of £15 million a year.

And in November 1986 Mr Philip Hunt, Director of the National Association of Health Authorities, told a seminar on security that crime could be costing the NHS £36 million a year. Mr Hunt said that in the North-west of England health-service equipment had, for example, turned up in junk shops, while runner beans were growing on crutches, and bedpans were being used as plant pots.

From my own experiences I suspect that the total amount of money lost to the NHS through dishonesty is far more than £36 million. More and more doctors are cheating the NHS by claiming money for work they have not done and in hospitals consultants (particularly surgeons) turn a blind eye to porters stealing linen because they are themselves busy stealing instruments and drugs for use on their private patients.

I estimate that in some areas between twenty-five and fifty per cent of the surgical equipment found in operating theatres in private hospitals will have been bought with NHS money.

WASTEFUL PRACTICES

For over a century the operating theatre ritual has included the wearing of masks in the theatre. The assumption is that masks are essential for preventing the contamination of wounds. But in 1982 a report published in an English surgical journal and written by Neil W. M. Orr of Colchester showed that when no masks were worn by anyone in the operating theatre the incidence of wound infections did not increase. In fact, the incidence of wound infections actually fell. The study involved one operating theatre and 432 separate wounds.

Also in 1982, a report from two surgeons at the Leicester Royal Infirmary, published in the *Lancet*, showed that the wearing of sterile surgical gloves by Casualty Unit staff did not decrease the rate of infection after wounds were repaired.

The two surgeons conducted a trial in their accident and emergency unit in which 418 wounds were sutured by nurses. In half of the cases the nurses wore gloves. In the other half the nurses did not wear gloves. All the wounds were sutured in the same way.

The surgeons concluded that if wounds were handled gently, and cleaned thoroughly, wound infection would remain low. Surgical gloves were irrelevant.

In August 1985 Mr Graham Barker, a senior registrar in obstetrics and gynaecology at the Middlesex Hospital in London published a report showing that swabbing the skin before giving injections is a waste of time and money.

Barker quoted several scientific reports which showed that there was no evidence to suggest that sterilizing the skin with alcohol swabs made any difference to the incidence of infection. The first of the papers showing that routine swabbing of the skin is unnecessary had been published back in 1969. Barker pointed out that his hospital alone used 800,000 swabs a year – at a cost (in 1985) of more than £3,000 per annum.

It is difficult to estimate how much money could be saved by abandoning surgical masks, not using surgical gloves during routine casualty-department suturing and abandoning the practice of swabbing areas of skin before giving injections. But the total saving must certainly be measured in millions of pounds each year.

UNNECESSARY DENTAL SURGERY

In 1984 the Junior Trade Minister, John Butcher, called for an enquiry into how two dentists in his Coventry constituency had managed to gross a million pounds in a single year while working in the NHS. Both the dentists had luxury homes. One had a forty-five-foot yacht moored on the coast of the south of France.

'It is extremely easy just to drill teeth needlessly and put in fillings that are larger than they need to be,' said Brian Lux, a member of the General Dental Council and a council member for the General Dental Practitioners' Association. Mr Lux pointed out that a small filling on a biting surface earns a dentist less than half as much as a filling that is extended to the front and back of the tooth.

By February 1986 the enquiry had made its report and it recommended tough sanctions to stop dentists from carrying out unnecessary treatment. The report said that in 1984 more than 280 dentists had gross earnings of over £100,000 but it went on to say that it was difficult to decide whether there was a correlation between very high earnings and unnecessary treatment. The British Dental Association said that it was heartened by the findings that the vast majority of dentists were not undertaking unnecessary treatment. It wholeheartedly supported the recommendations.

The 'tough' sanctions recommended by the official enquiry included:

- 'ensuring that all dental staff at the Dental Estimates Board should continue to attend regular refresher courses'

- 'arranging regular policy meetings between professional staff'

- 'not changing the definition of dental fitness'

- 'telling the Health Education Council to encourage patients to continue to visit the same dentist regularly for as long as they found him or her satisfactory'

By February 1987 things were moving fast. Mrs Edwina Currie, Parliamentary Secretary for Health, announced the Government's intention to implement the recommendations of the Committee of Enquiry into Unnecessary Dental Treatment. In answer to a parliamentary question Mrs Currie said that she was pleased to announce that thirty-two of the Committee's fifty-two recommendations 'have been or are in the process of being implemented. Active discussions are taking place about the implementation of a further fifteen.' She also announced that a committee had begun work to consider methods by which the Dental Estimates Board could be assisted in the assessment of the need for orthodontic treatment. Dishonest dentists all over Britain must have trembled at these proposals.

UNNECESSARY AND CUMBERSOME GP ADMINISTRATION

The massive bureaucratic machine which I have already described does not look after GPs, dentists or opticians. To 'manage' these independent providers of health care there are separate administrative entities: the Family Practitioner Committees.

The FPCs report directly to the DHSS in London. One of their main functions is to arrange for patients' notes to move about the country as patients themselves move from one area to another and, inevitably, change GPs. This simple administrative task is not managed with too much efficiency.

When a friend of mine recently moved house she, her husband, and their two children didn't move far – only about 100 miles or so. But six months after they had moved house their medical records still hadn't managed to reach their new GP.

In my friend's case the delay was inconvenient rather than dangerous. But in many instances such lengthy delays can prove disastrous. After all, when a patient suffers from a long-term problem such as diabetes, high blood pressure, epilepsy or asthma then it is absolutely vital that his medical records are always readily available.

Without access to previous medical records a doctor will find it difficult to treat any patient safely and effectively. He will have to start his medical treatment programme from scratch. And there will, inevitably, be a lot of unnecessary and potentially dangerous guesswork.

My friend's experience was not, however, unusual. According to the latest available figures it now takes an average of seventeen weeks for an envelope containing a patient's medical records to be moved from the patient's old doctor to his new one. It is by no means uncommon for the transfer to take more than twice that long.

It is worth looking at what happens. When a new patient is accepted by a GP, the doctor sends a completed form along to his local Family Practitioner Committee. The FPC then tells the administrators who look after the NHS Central Register and these administrators get in touch with the previous doctor's FPC. That Committee then gets in touch with the patient's former doctor and asks for the medical records. The records are then posted from the patient's former doctor to his FPC, from them to the new doctor's FPC, and from there on to the patient's new doctor. It is an unnecessarily cumbersome procedure. The administrators who are involved are quite unnecessary.

FPCs are desperately overstaffed with well-paid people who have nothing to do but shuffle pieces of paper around. In order to make their work look worthwhile they have to work slowly. Millions of pounds could be saved by sacking all FPC employees instantly.

And the medical records? Well, the easiest solution would be to give them to patients to take with them to their new home.

Alternatively the patient's new doctor could send a requisition form to the patient's old doctor and the patient's old doctor could post the medical records directly to the patient's new doctor. There would be no extra work for the GPs (they have to put the records in the post anyway). The administrative middlemen would have been completely cut out.

CLEANING, CATERING, AND LAUNDRY

In 1982 a Parliamentary Social Services Committee produced a report which suggested that £200 million could be saved by contracting much of the catering and cleaning in NHS hospitals out to private enterprise.

The report pointed out that over a third of the cost of running our hospitals was spent on catering, domestic services, laundry, portering, and building maintenance.

One private contractor thought that the estimate of £200 million was too low. He thought that £300 million could easily be saved. In Yorkshire, for example, one hospital alone saved itself £100,000 a year by having its cleaning done privately. There are 2,600 NHS hospitals.

By March 1987 the NHS had still only managed to save £86 million by introducing competitive tendering and by contracting out cleaning and laundry services. Three-quarters of that saving had been produced by hospitals themselves cutting down in anticipation of competitive tenders being submitted by private firms.

It had, therefore, taken five years to obtain less than half of the saving that had been predicted in 1982. Allowing for inflation an annual saving of at least £250 million should now be possible. This means that we are currently wasting £164 million on NHS cleaning and laundry services.

OTHER POTENTIAL SAVINGS

Every few months doctors', politicians', and patients' organizations make suggestions as to how money could be saved within the NHS. Few of these suggestions or proposals are acted upon, although most of them are sensible and practical.

Here are just a few of the recent examples of waste within the NHS – together with some suggestions as to how savings could easily be made:

- In a survey of GPs' habits (based on a Manchester study of 200 doctors' workloads – and quoted in the medical newspaper *General Practitioner* in November 1985) it was shown that while some GPs referred one in fifty of their patients to hospital others referred one in four of their patients to hospital. These enormous variations are not explicable in clinical terms. They must inevitably lead to an enormous amount of waste in terms of specialists' time and hospital facilities. Those GPs who refer one in four of their patients to hospital are probably in need of concentrated postgraduate training.

- A report on NHS transport showed that many NHS vehicles do no more than 200 miles a week and stand idle for five and a half days out of seven. In some areas twice as many drivers are employed as there are vehicles available. Health authorities with vehicle fleets pay full, 'high street' prices for spare parts and repair work. In one city it was shown that two health authorities were using the same taxi firm to transport staff and patients. One authority paid rates twenty-two per cent higher than the other. According to this report at least one-quarter of the 6,000 health-authority vehicles are surplus to requirements. The transport study, published by the DHSS in 1984, concluded that some NHS staff spend up to forty per cent of their working week driving and that there are probably 20,000 NHS staff members who travel more than 5,000 miles a year on official duty – most of whom are paid on a mileage basis.

- Mr Kevin Short, district administrative officer for the Newry and Mourne area in Northern Ireland, admitted that changing a light bulb in an NHS hospital can cost over £30. Only qualified electricians are allowed to change light bulbs and in some hospitals two men must work together. If there is no electrician on call in a hospital, then an electrician may have to travel many miles from another institution.

- In 1985 Coventry and Warwickshire Hospital in Coventry appealed for accident victims to bring back crutches and walking sticks that they had been lent. The Deputy Hospital Administrator pointed out that crutches cost £11 a pair and sticks are £4 each. Apparently no record had been kept of patients who had been lent walking-sticks and crutches. (It is also worth noting that walking-sticks can be bought for less than £4 each. The hospital must have been buying them from a very expensive supplier.)

- Mrs Nora Saddington, a nursing director, was forced to take early retirement from the NHS when her £17,500 a year job disappeared in a Health Service reorganization. Mrs Saddington 'retired' in 1986. In March 1987 she was expected to earn £40,000 a year working as a private consultant to the NHS.

- In 1984 Mr Kenneth Clark, the Health Minister at the time, reported that the NHS loses about £10 million every year because health authorities fail to charge road accident victims, private patients, and overseas visitors (as they are entitled to under current regulations).

- Mr Jack Stockdale, Research Director of World Medical Markets, produced a report in 1983 showing that one in every twenty-two people was directly or indirectly employed by the NHS. Mr Stockdale showed that many companies supplying the NHS had been on an approved list since 1948 – and that no controls were exercised over their prices. Mr Stockdale estimated that if the supply monopoly were broken, the NHS would save between £40 million and £50 million a year.

- Nurses in the NHS change over 43 million nappies a year – 3,000 in the average maternity hospital each week. Cotton nappies cost 55 pence each and last for 200 washes at 11 pence a wash. Disposable nappies cost 5 pence each. The NHS could save £2 million a year by using disposable nappies.

- The NHS is one of the biggest property and landowners in Britain. In England it owns 50,000 acres of land – in addition to hospitals, health centres, clinics, offices, and staff accommodation. No attempts have been made to check that all this land is necessary or that it is being used effectively or efficiently. In 1985 it was estimated that the NHS owned over 100,000 houses, flats, and bedsitters. The estimate was made by Mr Fowler, Secretary of State for Social Services. According to the DHSS some health authorities have one-fifth of their accommodation standing empty.

- An independent report on non-emergency ambulance services, carried out under the supervision of Mr James Ackers, Chairman of the West Midlands Regional Health Authority, showed that £10 million a year could be saved. The report was published in 1984. No action has yet been taken. In 1981 another report showed that more than half the 999 calls made to the ambulance service are unjustified. No one knows how much a single ambulance call costs. No action was taken to reduce the abuse of the 999 ambulance service.

- Southampton surgeon Mr James Smallwood has reported that much of the blood ordered from central blood banks is poured down the drain. Mr Smallwood carried out an audit of the blood bank in the Portsmouth group of hospitals and reported that blood was unnecessarily cross-matched for operations and then thrown away if it wasn't used.

- A parliamentary select committee has reported that the NHS could save more than £60 million a year by buying more of its supplies in bulk. The All Party Public Accounts Committee said that the DHSS accepted that the savings could be made but that little had been done. The NHS spent about £1,700 million on non-medical supplies in 1981–2 (figures for the NHS are always very late in appearing). Few stores are bought in 'bulk'. In one region hospital stores and supplies are stored in fifty separate depots.

- There are virtually no controls on the buying of 'small' pieces of medical equipment. Surgeons order whatever they fancy. Much of this equipment goes to waste. Unnecessary supplies such as surgical instruments are frequently ordered on whims or in order to please or get rid of sales representatives. There are no controls within the NHS on the ordering of disposable equipment or equipment for use on the wards or in the operating theatre.

- In 1983 Chris Adams, Senior Consultant in Neurosurgery at the Radcliffe Hospital in Oxford, admitted in an interview printed in the *Daily Telegraph* that 'surgeons and physicians want the latest thing so that they can say they're one up on their friends down the road. Being well equipped is a boost to the ego. If people are honest, there is no doubt that a lot of new equipment is either wasted or underused.' Adams himself admitted that he had an ultrasonic aspirator which 'wasn't absolutely essential' but which 'made life easier in a few cases each year'. The aspirator had cost between £50,000 and £60,000. He also told the *Daily Telegraph* that some years ago a colleague had installed a tent for operations but had then found that he couldn't use his microscope inside it. Adams subsequently bought the plastic screens for his cucumber frames.

- In 1986 it was reported by the DHSS that NHS hospitals had an annual fuel and power bill totalling £325 million. It was estimated by Ray Whitney, then Parliamentary Secretary for Health, that thirty per cent of this sum could be saved. This would pay for the cost of building four general hospitals a year. In addition it was reported that nearly half of this sum – £50 million – could be saved simply by increasing the awareness and commitment of staff. (In other words by persuading staff to turn down heating and turn off lights when they weren't needed.)

- In 1986 Brigadier Freddie Lucas resigned his £33,000-a-year post as General Manager of Birmingham Central Health Authority. Mr Lucas resigned after submitting a report highlighting widespread financial incompetence. He claimed that money was 'pouring through holes in the bucket'. Brigadier Lucas said that he was rendered impotent by 'pseudo general managers'.

- Also in 1986 Victor Paige, hired at £70,000 a year to run the NHS, resigned after eighteen months. He will probably be remembered for the fact that although he was employed to cut waste, his main action was to hire more administrators.

- According to 1984 figures up to £20 million of NHS money is used to provide loans for NHS staff to buy motor cars.

- Following the 1982 reorganization of the NHS an early retirement scheme was introduced. The scheme was expected to cost £8,600,000. Instead it cost £54 million and there were 2,830 premature retirements instead of the forecast 435. But many of the administrators who had retired were subsequently found work in another part of the NHS. At the end of the reorganization the number of administrators had actually risen by several thousand! Some administrators received severance payments of £20,000 but were reappointed within months.

- The 'Rayner Scrutiny Report', published in 1985, showed that the NHS is wasting several million pounds a year on unnecessary forms. According to the Rayner Report the NHS could save £4 million a year, plus a one-off saving of £4.4 million by cutting back on the number of forms. Rayner found that each of the 192 District Health Authorities in Britain uses about 1,200 different types of forms – many of which duplicate one another or are simply unnecessary. Additional savings could be made in production and storage procedures – not to mention the time spent filling in unnecessary forms.

- In 1987 it was reported that more than half of 1,000 circulars issued to health authorities by the DHSS were out of date. Some dated from 1947 – before the NHS started. Mr Fowler, Secretary of State for Social Services, said that 531 circulars had been cancelled.

- Drug companies which supply the NHS have a government-guaranteed profit margin of 17.9 per cent. Purchase of pharmaceuticals costs the NHS £1,500 million a year. Drug companies make bigger profits than most other companies.

- In January 1987 the NHS was urged to strive for better value for the £700 million a year it spends on professional and technical staff. A report by Sir Gordon Downey, Comptroller and National Auditor General, showed that some areas of the country employ up to sixty-four occupational therapists for every 100,000 people. Other areas make do with five. Sir Gordon pointed out that between 1976 and 1984 there had been a thirty-seven per cent increase in professional and technical staff. The report also said that it had been difficult to get the right number of physiotherapists and radiographers because the number of students was fixed by the cash available locally rather than by the needs of the NHS.

These are just some of the ways in which money is wasted in the NHS. There are many more. Not many years ago a pool of secretaries dealt with letters dictated by hospital consultants. Now most consultants have their own secretaries even though there is rarely enough work for them to do. The waste is enormous, often engendered by greed, dishonesty, ego, and sheer incompetence.

The waste is crippling the NHS and is responsible for the shortages and problems which result in thousands of unnecessary deaths every year.

All this is truly a scandal of horrifying proportions.

POSTSCRIPT – PRIVATE MEDICINE

For some years now private medicine has been one of the biggest growth industries in Britain. Huge private hospitals have sprung up all over the country and membership of private medical insurance schemes is one of the most popular perks for everyone in industry. Whether they spend their money directly (as cash) or indirectly (by having health insurance as part of their salary) millions of people spend hundreds of millions of pounds on buying private medical treatment.

Some people undoubtedly buy private medical treatment purely to avoid long waiting lists. (And there is good evidence to show that they are spending their money wisely – private patients do get seen more quickly than NHS patients.) But many people pay the exorbitant fees charged by private hospitals and private insurance companies because they assume that the quality of care will be better. They are wrong.

If you go into a private hospital, you'll almost certainly get a private room, your own television set, carpets on the floor and access to a telephone. You'll have much better food than patients get in NHS hospitals. And the medical and nursing staff may well treat you with more respect. But the quality of care you receive will be *lower* in a private hospital than it will be in an NHS hospital.

Here are three specific examples of the ways in which the quality of medical care in a private hospital is likely to be inferior.

First, if you go into an NHS hospital you will almost certainly be seen by at least one doctor every day. In practice you'll probably be seen by several doctors several times. And there will always be doctors resident in the hospital. If you fall ill during the middle of the night or at the weekend there will be a doctor on call who can be at your bedside within minutes. If you go into a private hospital, however, you may well go for several days without being seen by any doctors at all. And private hospitals don't usually have resident medical staff. If you fall ill during the middle of the night or at the weekend there may well be a delay of some hours before a doctor can be found.

Second, if you go into an NHS hospital the doctors and nurses looking after you will have access to some of the most sophisticated medical equipment in the world. And if the specialist looking after you doesn't have something he needs, then he will be able to refer you to a specialist elsewhere (in theory at least). In a private hospital, however, the specialist will not have access to such a wide range of important and potentially life-saving equipment. And he certainly won't find it as easy to refer you to a specialist working in a better-equipped NHS hospital.

Third, if you are in an NHS hospital and you are unhappy about the treatment you are receiving then there are efficient and well-designed complaints procedures for you to use. A word to the ward sister or hospital administrator will usually ensure that your complaint receives attention. Should you be in a private hospital, however, there are unlikely to be any official complaints procedures. Indeed, if you are a patient in a private hospital and you are dissatisfied with the quality of care you receive there is almost certain to be nothing that you can do about it. The DHSS has admitted that 'there is little the Department can do for individuals who are dissatisfied with medical treatment obtained at a private establishment . . . the Department has no power to intervene'. And there is no point in hoping that your medical insurers will stand by you. Insurance organizations insist that they have no responsibility for the quality of care provided.

These are just three of the reasons why I think that many patients who pay for private treatment get worse medical care than they would have received inside the NHS; three of the reasons why I think that paying to go private is a waste of money; and three of the reasons why a growing number of practising doctors now insist that if they are taken ill they would prefer to go into an old-fashioned dingy, inefficient NHS ward.

The NHS reeks of inefficiency and waste. But exactly the same wasteful procedures are employed within the private health sector. There are few advantages – but many disadvantages – to going private.

SCANDAL No. 7

Inequalities in Health Care

It is called a National *health service. And inasmuch as the rules and regulations which govern the provision of health services are the same from Kent to Cumbria there is some justification for the name. But the quality or quantity of services available varies enormously from one part of the country to another.*

As far as the NHS is concerned, Britain is divided into sixteen separate regions (Scotland, Wales, and fourteen Regional Health Authorities in England). The quality of care you enjoy depends very much upon which region you happen to live in. And there aren't just subtle variations in hospital-building programmes – there are extremely vital variations in the type of care available and the length of time you're likely to have to wait in order to get treated. Where you live can have a very real influence on whether you live or die.

The facilities available to patients vary enormously from one part of the country to another.

Not long ago the parents of a young boy who needed laser surgery struggled to raise thousands of pounds to send their son to America. No surgeon in their part of the country had access to the equipment their son needed. The consultant they saw told them that if they could get their son to America, find the money for the journey, the accommodation, the specialist, and the hospital care he needed, then it might be possible to save his life. What neither they nor their consultant knew was that there was an NHS surgeon in the North-east of England who was an established world authority on laser surgery. He had done over one hundred operations of the type the small boy needed.

For me that case highlighted the little-known fact that the quality of service available within the NHS varies enormously from one town to another. Not even medical experts in Britain can keep up with what their colleagues across the country are doing.

If you break a limb and your bones refuse to mend and you live in a

145

village in the north of Scotland or the wilds of Cornwall, then you'll probably just have to put up with the pain and wait for a miracle. But if you have exactly the same problem and you just happen to live near to the Royal Hallamshire Hospital in Sheffield then you'll probably be able to see a consultant orthopaedic surgeon who has pioneered a new technique for encouraging rapid bone repair – using special electrical treatment to stimulate the healing process.

If you are involved in a road accident which results in an arm or leg being severed, then try to make sure that the accident happens in Lancashire. The Withington Hospital in Manchester is probably one of the best places to go to with that sort of problem. There, a team of consultant surgeons has developed microsurgery techniques which enable limbs to be sewn on that have been completely cut off.

Should your liver start to fail there isn't usually much that your doctor can do, unless he knows the specialized centres in which liver transplantation is regularly carried out in Britain. For example, they have done a large number of such operations at Addenbrooke's Hospital in Cambridge (though whether or not such operations are a worthwhile way to spend NHS money is another matter altogether – see page 159).

The variations around the country are enormous. At the Cardio-thoracic Institute, linked to the University of London, doctors have developed a nuclear-powered pacemaker that is fuelled by pluto-nium. There is a surgeon at King's College Hospital in London who has performed operations on unborn babies. There are doctors at University College Hospital, London, who use a laser for treating peptic ulcers. There are facilities in Manchester for helping infertile couples have a test-tube baby on the health service. There are special 'pain clinics' in some health service hospitals where patients can borrow TENS machines.

A technique which may be taken for granted in one hospital may be unheard of somewhere else. And a piece of equipment used regularly at one hospital may be nothing more than an entry in an illustrated catalogue at another hospital.

But important though these differences may be they are only a small part of the story. What I find even more worrying is the fact that there are, around the country, enormous variations in the way that common ailments are treated.

So, for example, if you are waiting to have your gall bladder removed and you live in the West Midlands, then you'll probably have to wait twice as long as you would if you lived in London. If you want an abortion, you'll stand a much better chance of having it done on the health service if you live in the North-western Region than if you live in the Yorkshire Region.

If you live in South Tees, fifty-three per cent of non-urgent general surgical cases have been on the waiting list for over a year. In North Tees, next door, no patients have been waiting over a year. Similarly, in South Manchester thirty-two per cent of patients waiting for non-urgent general surgery have been waiting for over a year, while in North Manchester no patients have been waiting over a year.

If you want to see a dentist and you live in the north of England, you'll find it nearly twice as difficult to find a dental surgery as you would if you lived in the South-east. If you need to have an operation on your hip, then you may have to wait ten, twenty or even a hundred times as long as your cousin who lives just fifty miles away.

And, of course, these variations are constantly changing. By the time you read this the Yorkshire Region may be the best place in Britain to have an abortion done and the waiting list for gall-bladder operations in London may exceed the waiting list for the same operation in the West Midlands.

As I write, the waiting list for heart surgery is five times as long in the North Region as it is in the Wessex Region and the waiting list for a piles operation is on average four times as long in Nottingham as it is in Liverpool.

These variations don't just affect surgery. There are similar differences in the waiting times for patients requiring admission to hospital for medical problems. If you live in the Yorkshire Region and you need a bed for an elderly relative, you'll be pleased to know that there are 10.4 beds available for patients over sixty-five years for every 1,000 members of the population. But in the North-west Thames Region there are only 6.6 geriatric beds for each 1,000 people. There are rather more than 20,000 fully fledged GPs in Britain. In the West Midlands or the North-west more than fifteen per cent of all GPs have over 3,000 patients to look after. In the South-east such overcrowding is very uncommon.

These enormous variations in health-service facilities are more than unfair. They have a dramatic effect on the quality of health care in different parts of the country. In Yorkshire fifteen out of every 1,000 babies die before they reach their first birthday. In East Anglia eleven out of every 1,000 babies die before they reach their first birthday. By and large people who live in the prosperous South-east are far more likely to enjoy a long life and good health than people who live in the north of England or Scotland. If you just happen to live in a region where facilities are well run and where essential services get priority, then you'll stand a much better chance of living to collect your pension.

But it gets worse. There aren't only huge differences between waiting times for essential, life-saving surgery in different regions, there are also very considerable differences within local areas, and even between consultants working in the same hospital. For example, I recently managed to get hold of a confidential list of waiting times for surgeons and physicians working in a large city in the midlands. The list shows quite dramatically how waiting times can vary enormously between hospitals that are only a matter of yards away from one another and between consultants actually working in the same hospital.

For example, the shortest length of time you'd have to wait if your GP referred you to Skin Specialist A was five weeks. If your GP referred you to Skin Specialist B in the same hospital, you'd have to wait thirty-two weeks for your first appointment.

If your daughter needed to have her tonsils removed and your GP referred her to Ear Nose and Throat Surgeon A, then she would have to wait three weeks for an appointment. If your GP referred her to Ear Nose and Throat Surgeon B at a nearby hospital then the wait would be sixty-two weeks.

If you needed to have a hip operation and required an appointment with an orthopaedic surgeon, the waiting time with surgeon A would be about one month. If you had an appointment with surgeon B at the same hospital – working in the same clinic but on different days of the week – then the waiting time for an initial appointment would be a massive thirty-one months – two and a half years.

Of all the health-service inequalities which exist it is probably these differences in waiting times for hospital appointments and for hospital admission which cause the greatest confusion, concern and distress. I have already pointed out elsewhere in this book that I believe that much medical and surgical treatment is unnecessary and more likely to do harm than good. But there are times when medical or surgical treatment is needed – and will help ease a patient's symptoms or improve his life expectation. And when treatment is necessary then a lengthy waiting time can be, to say the least, frustrating. It can also lead to unnecessary pain and, in a good many cases, to an early and possibly unnecessary death.

For some years now the number of patients on waiting lists in Britain has hovered between 600,000 and 800,000 although there is real evidence to show that the genuine figure is much higher than this. In May 1987 the College of Health reported that 'some patients have to wait four years or more for treatment and others are dying before their turn comes'. According to the College of Health seventy per cent of patients needing urgent treatment fail to get it within a month.

In October 1986 the *British Medical Journal* published an article entitled 'DHSS Waiting-List Statistics – A Major Deception' written

148

by P. A. Sykes, a consultant surgeon at Park Hospital in Manchester. Sykes points out that when collecting statistics about waiting lists the DHSS instructs its staff to exclude various categories of patients. The excluded groups include day cases, patients who wish to defer admission for personal reasons and patients who do not require admission until a later date for a medical reason – for example, patients who need to lose weight before surgery or patients waiting for additional operations or for cataract surgery.

Sykes also notes that the presentation of official DHSS waiting lists is misleading. The DHSS, he reports, records only the number of patients waiting for admission in each speciality and does not allow for the expected time in hospital for each patient.

But the main problem that Sykes identifies is the exclusion of some patients who need treatment, who are waiting for treatment but who, for administrative reasons, are not counted.

Sykes concludes that the true number of patients awaiting admission to hospital is 79.9 per cent greater than the official figure.

If these figures are accepted (and Mr Sykes' conclusions have not been disputed by the DHSS), then there are in truth well over 1 million people in Britain currently waiting to be admitted to hospital.

The real scandal here is, I believe, the fact that waiting lists are largely unnecessary; they exist not because of any genuine shortage of facilities or specialists but because of incompetence and inefficiency and because consultants actually like having long waiting lists.

There are, I believe, several explanations for our enormous national waiting list. First, there is the undoubted fact that many patients are put on to the waiting list quite unnecessarily. As I have already shown in this book (see page 62), many patients have operations which they do not need.

Second, there is the fact that different specialists keep patients in hospital for different lengths of time for exactly the same procedure. A few years ago, for example, a study was performed to investigate the amount of time men spent in hospital after having elective hernia repair operations. The hernia repair operation was chosen because it is a relatively standard surgical procedure. The survey involved eight hospitals and nine consultant surgeons. All the hospitals were in the south of England. Just over 1,000 patients aged between sixteen years and sixty-five years were included in the survey. The survey showed that after their operations the men spent between one and twenty-three days in hospital. The average length of time spent in hospital after surgery was 5.7 days but the mean for each of the eight hospitals varied between 3.8 days and 9.3 days.

There is absolutely no logical explanation for these differences. It is logical that an occasional patient will develop complications and will need to stay in hospital for longer. But a hernia repair operation is a hernia repair operation and the only reason why there could be such huge differences between the *average* amounts of time spent in hospital is incompetence. Either the surgeons involved or the hospitals involved were guilty of gross professional incompetence.

Since the study also showed that when the surgeons involved operated at more than one hospital it was the hospital not the surgeon that influenced length of stay the conclusion has to be that in this particular example it was incompetence within the hospital that was responsible for the unnecessarily lengthy stays.

And there is other evidence to support this conclusion. A report published by the Office of Health Economics in 1982 showed that long waiting lists are caused overwhelmingly by deficiencies in waiting-list management. In addition, however, the report showed that few hospitals are operating at the limit of their physical capacity. Most operating theatres in British hospitals have an average working time of thirty-seven weeks a year – predominantly because of lost sessions due to Bank Holidays. And even during those thirty-seven weeks the operating theatres are used relatively sparingly. The report pointed out that because of shortage of staff in the evening, 'it is frequently difficult for a surgeon to start an operation after 4.30 p.m.' So if an operation ends at that sort of time, the operating theatre will simply close down.

In 1985 evidence came to light that made British hospitals look even worse than this. Mr John Yates of the Health Services Management Centre at Birmingham University concluded that empty beds, wasted operating theatres, and reluctant surgeons were key causes of long National Health Service waiting lists. 'It seems an incredible paradox,' concluded Mr Yates, 'that we should have 50,000 acute beds, one-quarter of the total, empty each day.'

In an article in the *National Association of Health Authorities' Newsletter* Yates pointed out that there are wide variations in how efficiently beds are used in each health authority. For example, on average, forty-three per cent of ear, nose and throat beds were empty each day. Yates also said that he had evidence that many surgeons were unwilling to operate. 'I have,' he said, 'found examples of surgeons who have only been given one operating session a week despite being on a full-time contract.'

Even more recently other evidence has shown that things in British hospitals are, if anything, getting worse not better. An article in the medical newspaper *GP* in July 1986 reporting that a common reason for long waiting lists is inefficiency, pointed out that 'there is wide acceptance that the running of the operating theatres in many hospitals is spectacularly mismanaged'. A study in one unidentified region revealed that on any one day half the theatres were empty.

An investigation in Oxford confirmed these almost unbelievable findings. The study there showed that the main problems were that a quarter of the operating theatre sessions were unallocated and that a third of those that were held finished early. In addition the average operating session started sixteen minutes late.

(An article in the *British Medical Journal* in early 1987 provided additional confirmation. The article was written by an anaesthetist who complained that operating sessions rarely started on time since surgeons were invariably late in arriving for work.)

But incompetence and inefficiency aren't the only reasons for long waiting lists. There is, of course, also the problem that at least a tenth of our hospital beds are, at any one time, occupied by patients who have been made ill by doctors' treatments. Patients who suffer drug side effects or who develop complications after surgery have to be kept in hospital for longer periods. The more incompetent a surgeon, the longer his patients will spend in hospital.

And hospital infections are beginning to play an increasingly important part in the development of waiting lists, too. Roughly five per cent of all hospital patients acquire infections while in hospital which are so bad that they need to stay in hospital for, on average, an extra four days.

Finally, there is the fact that a good many consultants (and this is particularly true of surgeons) deliberately keep their waiting lists as long as possible. I can illustrate this best with a true anecdote.

Not long ago a friend of mine who is a surgeon took a job standing in for a surgical consultant who had gone abroad for three months. When he started work, my friend found that the surgeon had left him with a modest waiting list several months long. Without making any particular effort my friend found that by the time the consultant arrived home he had managed to reduce the waiting list to virtually nothing. He didn't work any faster than was safe, but the waiting list just melted away. Being rather naive my friend was rather proud of this. In his innocence he thought that the returning surgeon would be pleased. Not a bit of it. The consultant was furious. And he was furious for two reasons which he quickly explained – illustrating his explanation with a healthy variety of well-known expletives which I will, for the sake of good taste, delete from this account.

First, he explained to my friend, if he had no NHS waiting list, he could hardly expect to get any private patients. After all most patients who go private pay the money to get seen quickly. And second, he pointed out that in his opinion his status as a surgeon had been damaged. He believed that if GPs could send patients along to his clinic and expect them to be admitted to hospital without any delay, then they would have little regard for him. As far as he was concerned a long waiting list was a sign that he was held in high esteem.

After talking to a number of other hospital doctors I am convinced that those feelings are by no means unusual. And if you think that I am exaggerating let me make two small points.

First, hospital consultants who see private patients almost always have longer waiting lists than consultants who don't ever see any private patients. And second, whatever attempts are made to cut waiting lists they never change. The total number of people waiting for hospital treatment in Britain has been between 600,000 and 800,000 for as long as most people can remember.

Before I end this section there is one final explanation for our long waiting lists that cannot be ignored.

According to Sir Douglas Hague, Chairman of the Social Science Research Council, waiting lists are created by doctors who choose to do the things they are doing rather than the things they might be doing. For example, says Hague, they choose to do spectacular high-technology operations rather than getting rid of queues for hip-joint replacements and varicose-vein operations.

In private many consultants admit that this is right. One surgeon at a London teaching hospital has admitted that one of the reasons why there are especially long waiting lists for things like hernias and varicose veins is because they are boring operations to do. 'A lot of surgeons,' agreed a professor of surgery, 'would rather do one or two interesting operations than sixteen hernias.' I suspect that a lot of patients would find that attitude unacceptable.

On a purely practical level it is perhaps also worthwhile pointing out that hospital waiting lists have now been so outrageously long for such an enormous length of time that many advisers have come up with schemes for 'beating' the waiting lists. Obviously, the easiest technique is to go private. But paying for a full operation can be exceedingly costly and many patients simply cannot afford this sort of expenditure. In addition as I've already explained (see page 142) it is often better to go into an NHS hospital than into a private hospital. The answer, therefore, is to have an initial private consultation with a specialist and then to transfer to the NHS waiting list. This way for an outlay of perhaps £30 or so a patient gains time in two specific ways. First, his initial appointment will be much quicker. (The waiting time for a first appointment can be many months whereas the waiting time for private appointments is rarely longer than a couple of weeks.) Second, consultants who see patients privately often put them on to their more 'urgent' NHS waiting lists. This may be because the patient, having had longer to explain his problem, can persuade the specialist to be more sympathetic or it may be because the specialist feels that he 'owes' the patient a favour. Whatever the explanation the fact is that patients can benefit enormously by buying an initial private consultation and then having any essential treatment performed under the NHS.

SCANDAL No. 8

Confused Priorities

One of the biggest scandals in late twentieth-century medicine is the way that medicine has been allowed to develop without any logical plan. Money has been spent wildly on innovative and often imaginative research projects which can, at best, hope to help only a tiny minority of patients. On the other hand patients needing routine medical care have been abandoned to their fate.

Doctors hate thinking in terms of 'value for money'. Surgeons and physicians who have deliberately allowed long waiting lists to develop, and who have knowingly allowed patients to suffer unnecessarily, suddenly seem to become very concerned about the rights of their patients when economists and politicians start talking about the need to establish priorities in medicine.

What those doctors are really concerned about is, of course, their own professional status. No doctor, and in particular no specialist, likes to think of his department being run down or deprived of valuable resources. Specialists are not good at thinking in general, broad terms; they tend to see only their own limited aims and professional ambitions.

When the National Health Service began in 1948 it was believed that demand for health care would gradually fall. Nye Bevan and his colleagues who helped found the NHS firmly and honestly believed that their new scheme would gradually cure all illnesses and that the reduction in sickness and ill health would so improve the productivity of the nation that the cost of running the NHS would be negligible. They could not have been more wrong.

Over the years the demand for health care has steadily grown and as doctors and scientists have created new treatments and new diagnostic machinery so the need for money has grown too. Today we could easily spend our entire Gross National Product on health care. And there would still be long waiting lists for essential, boring operations. Money cannot solve our health service problems. The only real solution is for us to accept that there have to be priorities within the system.

Of course, in a rather haphazard way doctors have for decades been making choices about which patients to save and which patients to abandon. They have had to choose which patients to admit to hospital, which patients to operate on, and which patients to use as guinea pigs for new treatments. But doctors have never really examined the way in which they deploy their resources. They have always been unwilling to accept that they should try to be cost-effective.

Patients, too, have found the idea of there having to be choices in health care rather unacceptable. They have for decades been dazzled by new drugs, new equipment, and fantastic promises. They have been conned into believing that the sky is the limit as far as the healing power of modern medicine is concerned. Many people genuinely and honestly believe that the majority of killing and disabling diseases will, one day, be conquered. There is an implicit and unspoken belief in a medically inspired immortality.

The very idea that it may be necessary to make choices is something that most doctors and most patients have simply refused to accept.

When transplant operations were introduced into the NHS a few years ago no one really stopped to think how many patients would be deprived of more mundane operations in order to pay for the transplant technology. Countless expensive medical techniques have been brought into action without any attempt at evaluation. We have assumed that normal economic rules do not apply to the NHS. We have avoided such awful phrases as 'cost-effectiveness'.

And yet today, as we get closer and closer to the twenty first century, it becomes more and more obvious that the main constraints on health care are financial rather than medical or scientific. In the future our problems will not be what we can or cannot do, but what we can or cannot afford.

In fact, when you look back through history it becomes clear that this concept isn't really a new one. Back in 1876 it was suggested by a public-spirited French citizen that hand-operated ventilating machines should be placed at regular intervals along the banks of the Seine. These machines would, the citizen insisted, enable passers-by to revive unfortunate folk who had fallen into the river. The idea never became reality for the simple but important reason that it would have cost far too much money.

The real difference today is that we're spending far too much of our money on the late twentieth-century equivalent of the French ventilating machines.

155

It was, I suppose, the introduction of renal dialysis a few decades ago that really made it clear that the available financial resources cannot cope with the scientific possibilities. Within a short time of the first dialysis machine being produced doctors realized that they had to select patients to live and patients to die. They really did have the power of life or death. They simply could not afford to buy all the equipment they would need if they were to keep all such patients alive. Neither doctors nor patients found it easy to accept that resources had to be allocated according to need, effectiveness, and usefulness.

Associations representing specific groups of patients have fought hard for more money to spend on their own favourite project. And, of course, doctors have fought equally hard to obtain funds for their own personal research programmes. It has become commonplace for doctors to exaggerate their needs in order to arouse public sympathy and to force those who control the purse strings to disobey good sense and fund projects which may be of limited human value but which, nevertheless, have good 'media' potential. This type of activity is known in the profession as 'shroud waving' and you have only to open a popular newspaper to find yet another example.

As I write, I have a cutting in front of me which tells how a 'desperate doctor made a dramatic plea last night for £9,500 to save a young baby's life'. According to the newspaper the doctor needs the money to buy special chemicals in order to do diagnostic tests. 'We must have them in three or four days,' the doctor said. 'Without them the child will die.' On the television news last night there was a story about a young girl who will die if she doesn't have a liver transplant. The surgeon involved appeared on our screens telling us exactly what he needed.

It is no coincidence that these stories nearly always involve young children who are dying. Doctors know as well as journalists that these are the stories which will pull at the heart strings and produce the greatest impact, the greatest emotional appeal.

The problem is, of course, that 'shroud waving' distorts the whole picture yet again. 'Shroud waving' only helps the patients with dramatic problems. It only helps the doctors whose enthusiasms are for easily promotable aspects of high-technology medicine. It results in our valuable resources being divided among the most exciting aspects of hospital based high-technology medicine. The elderly, the mentally handicapped, the disabled, and the patients suffering from 'commonplace' disorders get very little.

I suspect that in the long run this scandal will do more harm than any other.

156

TRANSPLANTATION

Few subjects attract as much publicity as transplantation. I have a huge file of cuttings dealing with heart transplants, liver transplants, kidney transplants, and brain transplants. I have cuttings describing the first man to man transplant and the first operation which involved putting a monkey's heart into a man. I have stories of babies having complicated transplant operations and I have cuttings about a baby who received the heart of an animal. I have cuttings describing the world's first combined heart and lung transplant and I have cuttings which describe the transplantation of one animal's head on to another animal. To me it all seems vaguely obscene. I have several objections to transplant surgery.

My first objection is a straightforward ethical one. It is now over twenty years since I first appeared as a guest on a television programme. And I can still remember that programme very clearly. The main guest was Dr Christiaan Barnard – the man who had just performed the world's first heart-transplant operation. And the rest of us were there to question the rights and wrongs of it all.

Even then, way back in 1967, I was terrified of what transplant surgery might mean to our society. It was ethical fears which were uppermost in my mind, although at the time I was confused about exactly why I felt that it was wrong. Today those ethical fears are much clearer.

Before I go on let me just say that I can well understand why those whose friends or relatives who are waiting for transplant surgery feel so strongly about the whole subject. If I were in their shoes, I have absolutely no doubt that I would feel exactly the same as they do. If a member of my family were desperately ill and could only be saved by a transplant operation, I would fight tooth and nail for them to have such an operation. I would heartily oppose anyone who stood in my way. But in a way that is the major weakness of transplantation. It encourages a selfishness, an aggressiveness, and a kind of anti-social behaviour that, in the long run, can only lead to problems.

My main ethical objection to transplantation is that, although a code of practice has been prepared for transplant surgeons, the fact remains that when hearts and livers are taken from patients those hearts and livers must still be in good working order. They are, indeed, taken from patients who may be technically dead, but who are, in ordinary practical terms, very much alive. And I find that difficult to accept.

If you think that I'm making a fuss about nothing, then let me ask you a very simple question: If a relative of yours were lying in a hospital bed with his heart still beating and blood still flowing around his body would you give consent for his body to be buried if the surgeons told you that there was no hope?

If you would be happy to see your relative taken, with beating heart, and fed into the crematorium, then that is fine. You obviously don't have any qualms about the ethics of transplant surgery. But if you, like me, find this a repulsive and frightening thought then you have to ask yourself whether you could approve of surgeons removing the living heart from such a relative. Or anyone else, come to that. Of course, now that surgeons are beginning to experiment with transplanting bits and pieces of brain tissue the number of ethical problems will undoubtedly grow even faster.

My second objection to transplantation is that it exposes patients to a potentially horrifying experience that has little to do with medicine or ordinary health care. And here, to support my belief, I will quote experts who have far more experience of dealing with transplant patients than I have.

One of America's leading heart surgeons, Michael DeBakey, gave up heart transplantation entirely because 'the results obtained don't justify the sacrifices made'. While in England Dr Michael Petch, a cardiologist who worked as part of the Papworth Hospital transplant team from 1977 to 1980 withdrew for the simple but powerful reason that 'overall, the treatment was not sufficiently better than the disease'. Petch has described how, when he decided to withdraw from the transplant programme, he felt as if a burden had been lifted from his shoulders.

'All recipients have at least one complication,' wrote Petch in a thoughtful article written two years after leaving the Papworth programme. He then went on to point out that about a third of recipients die in the first year after transplantation. Petch has also pointed out that heart transplants at Papworth have inevitably interfered with the work of the hospital.

Other observers have also shown considerable distaste at the way that transplant patients have suffered. For example, Philip Blaiberg, Dr Barnard's most famous heart-transplant patient, who survived for eighteen months, had two severe bouts of heart failure, a severe episode of jaundice due to drugs, and meningitis due to lowered resistance to infection caused by the drugs he was taking to stop his body rejecting the heart he had been given.

Inevitably, since they and their patients are in the public eye, transplant surgeons do everything in their power to keep their patients alive. They strive officiously to maintain life even when that life is of doubtful value.

My third serious objection to organ transplantation is that it is extremely expensive. The cost of transplanting a heart (or indeed any other organ) from one patient to another is difficult to estimate accurately. But when capital costs are included it will be well over £20,000. And to that must be added the cost of continuing drug treatment – which can easily run into several thousand pounds a year. Every year in Britain 200,000 people die from heart disease. And most of them could be saved by transplants. Multiply 200,000 by £20,000 and the overall potential cost of transplant surgery becomes clear.

Those working in transplant units will undoubtedly disagree with my estimate. But they have a rather unusual way of managing their accounts. For example, in an article in *General Practitioner* in May 1987 Dr Nicholas Norwell, a GP in Berkshire, pointed out that when a patient of his had a transplant he received a letter from the transplant unit instructing him to send a prescription to the hospital for drugs that the patient required. When he telephoned the transplant unit Dr Norwell was told that 'if the unit could cut its drug bill by £20,000 a year it could perform an extra two transplants'. This sort of imaginative accounting doesn't help the NHS or its patients. It merely helps the transplant unit.

Inevitably, given the cost, there has to be a selection system. If you are a thirty-year-old woman with three children and an important job at the Regional Health Authority headquarters, then you will go to the top of the list if you need a transplant. But if you are a fifty-five-year-old woman with no dependents and no job, then your position on the list will be far less secure. And if you happen to annoy the transplant surgeon or if he arrives at the clinic in a bad temper, then there has to be a chance that there will be no room for you on the transplant programme.

This sort of selection system is clearly unacceptable. It is terribly unjust. And yet if transplant surgery is going to continue, then the selection system will have to stay. We will never, ever be able to afford to provide transplant operations for all those patients who may need them. The simple, unavoidable truth is that we have to have priorities. We have to try and spend our limited financial resources in such a way that the greatest number of patients benefit. And we have to forget the emotional arguments and the 'shroud waving' and try to make our decisions in a cool and clinical way.

The doctors who work in transplant surgery have one enormous advantage when it comes to campaigning for a bigger share of the NHS cake. They can point to individual lives that they have saved. They can photograph individuals whose lives can be saved. This sort of emotional blackmail is often very effective.

159

In the 1970s heart transplants were banned in Britain as a result of advice from the DHSS. Thousands of doctors had expressed doubt about the usefulness and ethical quality of this work. But the transplant surgeons fought hard for the right to resume their work. And they found it easy to harness public opinion behind them. The result was that in 1979, even though the major doubts about heart transplantation still had not been resolved, two heart-transplant programmes were reinstated.

Today the operation still has not been properly evaluated. There are still no rules about how patients will be chosen for surgery. And there is no real check on the way in which transplant programmes adversely affect other patients with simpler needs. The real scandal is that those surgeons who perform transplants are selecting individual patients to live and condemning thousands to death. I have no doubt that thousands of people who have died of heart disease in the last few years would still be alive today if the money spent on transplantation had been spent instead on preventive medicine. The simple fact is that most heart disease is preventable.

THE ULTIMATE CHOICE – THE LIFE OR DEATH DECISION

In 1985 Derek Sage, who had been receiving kidney dialysis at a large hospital outside London, was refused further treatment. The consultant in charge of the kidney unit said that the hospital had difficulty managing Sage because he was incontinent and abusive. Others confirmed that Sage was schizophrenic and mentally defective. He was also unemployed and rootless. His home was in a hostel. 'I don't see why once you have taken someone on for treatment you have to continue until he dies on the dialysis machine,' said the consultant afterwards, when questioned about his decision.

After an appeal that failed, Sage was discharged from hospital. Then, with the help of Mr Sage's GP and the British Kidney Patient Association (one of Britain's most vocal and persuasive pressure groups) Sage was found a place at a hospital in London.

Many other patients are not, of course, quite so lucky. Patients are refused dialysis for a variety of reasons. Age is one of the commonest reasons for refusing dialysis. Some doctors believe that any patient older than fifty who has kidney disease should be left to die. Other doctors believe that patients should be given dialysis up to the age of fifty-five. Patients have also been turned down for dialysis because they are disabled, because they are homeless, because they are diabetic, and because they don't speak English. One patient was, apparently, turned down because he had a neurotic wife.

Occasionally, there is a public outcry when a reporter hears that a particular patient has been refused access to a dialysis machine and has, effectively, been told to go away and die. But more often than not nothing happens. And in fact it is impossible to avoid the conclusion that having invented dialysis and having made it available within the NHS, we have created for ourselves a permanent problem. The plain truth is that if we spent our entire Gross National Product on dialysis machines we would never be able to provide dialysis for every patient needing it. Kidney dialysis may be a wonderful piece of high-technology medicine, but it has provided us with an insoluble moral problem. We now have the ability to keep people alive even though their kidneys do not function properly. But we cannot afford to keep all patients with malfunctioning kidneys alive. And so, as long as there are kidney dialysis machines, there will have to be choices. Patients will have to be selected to live or to die. The advocates of high-technology medicine have presented us with the most awesome of dilemmas.

THE FORGOTTEN MILLIONS

Test-tube babies cost the NHS millions of pounds. The cost of keeping one premature baby alive is estimated at £75,000. Heart and liver transplant programmes take millions of pounds of NHS money. And other high-technology 'experimental' programmes cost millions more. Savings have to be made somewhere.

One area where the DHSS has made most of its savings in the last ten years has been in the treatment of the mentally ill. For a decade now the official policy has been to try and close as many long-stay institutions as possible. Unlike some official programmes this one has been managed extremely effectively. In the last ten years the number of people resident in mental hospitals in Britain has fallen by a quarter. Officially, spokesmen for the DHSS claim that they are closing long-stay institutions so that more mentally ill patients can live constructive, rewarding lives in the community.

In theory the policy sounds very laudable. But in practice it is proving to be an absolute disaster and it is clear to most observers that the programme is designed not to help the mentally ill but to save money. The care of the mentally ill is not a priority in the NHS of the late 1980s. If mental hospitals were closing because patients were moving into the community I would cheer, but in practice patients are moving into the community because hospitals are closing. There is a big difference.

All over Britain thousands of mentally ill patients – many of whom have spent their lives in institutions of one sort or another, and who are not capable of looking after themselves – are being turned out into the streets. Britain has 160,000 severely intellectually handicapped and 500,000 mildly intellectually handicapped people. In addition there are approximately 500,000 schizophrenics in Britain. Some go and live in hostels where they are provided with dirty rooms and terrible food. They are thrown out after breakfast and not allowed back again until evening. Whatever the weather they must spend their days roaming the streets. Others, more fortunate, go and live with relatives. But only rarely is this a perfect solution. The arrival of a mentally retarded or unstable relative can totally disrupt a tightly knit household. Children have to be turned out of their bedrooms to make room for the newcomer. There isn't enough money to go round. Guilt and resentment quickly build to intolerable levels.

The main problem is that although the DHSS has been enthusiastically closing down mental hospitals and other long-stay institutions, it has done virtually nothing to help those patients settle into the community. Millions of pounds have been saved by closing down long-stay hospitals, but nothing has been spent on building day-care centres or sheltered workshops. Nothing has been spent on providing relatives with support and guidance. Thousands of patients who need more or less constant care and attention have been left to fend for themselves.

The reason is simple enough. Mental illness is not fashionable. There is no 'shroud waving' on behalf of schizophrenics. And the mentally ill have no political clout. They don't even have the vote.

SCANDAL No. 9

High-technology Preventive Medicine Doesn't Work – And Isn't Necessary

We know what causes eighty per cent of all cancers. We know what causes at least ninety per cent of all heart attacks. We know how high blood pressure – the main cause of strokes – can be controlled without drugs. We could, with a little effort and a modest but well-organized educational programme, prevent most cancers, most cases of heart disease and most strokes. But this simple solution does not appeal to health-care professionals. Doctors have always earned their living treating illness and they look down their noses at the practice of prevention. The huge, prosperous, and profitable health-care industry doesn't like the idea of illness being prevented without any opportunity for profit.

So, as a compromise, a new form of 'high-technology interventionist preventive medicine' has been designed. Patients who want to stay healthy and avoid disease are offered sophisticated screening programmes, vaccines, and other 'high-tech' solutions.

However, this new branch of medicine is not just unnecessary: it doesn't work. Preventive medicine – as practised in the 1980s – is a scandal.

The importance of keeping people healthy by teaching them how to regulate their lifestyles is well established. Over two thousand years ago Hippocrates advocated a regime of fresh air, exercise, good food, hydrotherapy, and massage. He knew the real value of preventive medicine. Through the centuries hundreds of other eminent authors have passed on the same message. Emile Zola summed up the value of prevention best in an anecdote about a physician who is so busy on the river bank fishing people out of the water that he has no time to go upstream to find out who is pushing them in.

It is not difficult to explain why, on economic, social and humanitarian grounds, it is better to spend money on preventive medicine than on almost any aspect of medical research or high-powered hospital medicine. We have over the last few years spent hundreds of millions of pounds searching for a magic cure for cancer. If we had spent the same amount of money on preventive medicine, there is no doubt that a large number – probably at least half – of the people who have cancer today would not have cancer.

We have spent millions on looking for treatments for heart disease. But if we had spent our money on education, on teaching people to eat the right foods, lose weight, stop smoking and take more exercise, then we would have cut the number of heart attacks by at least half. By using our resources more sensibly we could have prevented disease wholesale instead of offering retail medicine to patients already suffering. But preventive medicine has been undervalued, underestimated and underused.

Almost all the major causes of premature death are either created by environmental problems or are produced by bad habits. Stronger legislation, better marketing of advice, and more determined and aggressive programmes of education would have cut the British mortality and morbidity rates in half. If we had put more effort into preventing illness, we could have sacked every doctor in Britain and closed down the entire hospital service and still seen a massive improvement in the health of the nation.

In my book *The Story of Medicine* I showed how men like the nineteenth-century reformer Edwin Chadwick did far more good for the health of the British people than any dozen famous doctors. Diseases like tuberculosis, cholera, and typhoid were conquered not by physicians or surgeons but by journalists and politicians.

Preventive medicine has been consistently ignored or relegated to fourth division status within the world of medicine. There are, I believe, a number of reasons for this. First, there is no doubt that preventive medicine does not have the glamour or excitement to capture the public interest. Recognizing the need to 'personalize' medical stories newspaper and television journalists concentrate their efforts on stories which involve real, identifiable people. It is easy to produce drama from an operating theatre where a patient is being given a new heart. It combines all the elements which go to make a good news story. There is the skill of the surgeon, the wonder of science, and the smiling patient. It is less easy to get excited about a preventive medicine programme that will save 100,000 lives. It is easy to take a picture of a smiling young organ recipient and his family. But it is difficult to take a picture of 100,000 smiling young men and women who *won't* develop heart disease because of a disease-prevention campaign. Each one of the 100,000 who will be saved is just as real as the transplant recipient. But the idea is not anywhere near as easy to market.

The second reason why preventive medicine hasn't caught on is more sinister. As I have already explained earlier, our lives are constantly being manipulated by a huge number of people and organizations who are far less interested in our health than they are in our money. The companies who sell butter, tobacco, alcohol, and other killer products are desperately keen to keep to an absolute minimum the amount of money and effort that is spent on teaching us how to stay healthy. If we all *knew* the truth, if we *knew* how to stay healthy, then their profits would tumble.

The plain, undeniable truth is that not even the Government wants us to know how to stay healthy. Every year the Treasury receives over £9,000 million from the tobacco and alcohol industries alone. Without that money coming in income tax would have to rise to politically unacceptable levels. It is, perhaps, hardly surprising that the Government wants us to keep on smoking.

To this we must add the fact that the politicians are very well aware that if we cut the number of people dying from heart disease and cancer then our economic position will be even more precarious than it is at the moment. For example, a properly organized and efficient preventive medicine programme would result in far fewer people having heart attacks. The number of men dying in their forties would be cut dramatically. But such a change could produce financial problems for the Government. All those forty-year-old men who would have died will live to receive their pensions. They will put an even bigger strain on the country's annual budget.

Anyone who doubts my theory that the Government doesn't want preventive medicine campaigns to work should take a close, hard look at the way the only official preventive medicine group, the Health Education Council, has been treated.

For many years now the Health Education Council, financed by the Government but theoretically enjoying some independence, has produced leaflets and campaigns designed to persuade people to smoke less, eat less fat, and take more exercise. The Health Education Council has never really had much impact – largely because its campaigns have always been run in a rather patronizing, amateurish, schoolmasterly sort of way – but it has at least tried.

On several occasions during recent years the Health Education Council's attempts to wean us off our national diet of fags, booze and butter has drawn criticism from those parts of the Government and the civil service which have a primary allegiance to the industries making killer products. For example, the Ministry of Agriculture, Fisheries and Food (which is widely thought to be in the grip of the National Farmers' Union and the various food industry lobby groups) has consistently complained about the Health Education Council's attempts to persuade us to eat healthier food.

165

Ian Sutherland, a former Director of Education and Training for the Health Education Council, claims that he once attended a luncheon with the then chairman of the HEC at which they were 'asked by a minister and a member of parliament if the HEC could see its way to working with the sugar industry rather than against it'.

Eventually, in 1987, Norman Fowler, then Secretary of State for Social Services, announced that the Health Education Council was to be closed down and a new body, the Health Education Authority, was to take its place and its £10 million a year budget.

Naturally, the Government insisted that the new body would be just as independent as the Health Education Council. But many outside critics were more cynical and saw the change in the name and structure of the country's only official disease prevention programme as a sign that the Government had bowed to pressure from the tobacco, alcohol and food industries. Only time will tell just how independent the Health Education Authority will be. Personally, I will be surprised if it shows any signs of having teeth at all.

My cynicism about the new Authority is fuelled by the fact that the newly appointed deputy chairman of the Health Education Authority is a lady called Ann Burdus. Mrs Burdus is described as one of the most lively members of the new body. But she will only work part-time for the Health Education Authority. She works as a director of AGB, one of Europe's largest market-research companies. AGB carries out large-scale market research surveys for the tobacco, alcohol and food industries.

SCREENING PROGRAMMES – THE MEDICAL SOLUTION TO DISEASE PREVENTION

History contains a thousand lessons to show that doctors can do a tremendous amount of good simply by advising their patients to change their lifestyles. But few doctors have shown any enthusiasm for simple health education. Most have tried to turn preventive medicine into a new medical speciality. Instead of teaching patients how to look after themselves and how to spot the early signs of illness (there is a wonderfully appropriate old Chinese saying which goes: if you give a man a fish you feed him for a day, if you teach him how to fish you feed him for a lifetime) doctors have concentrated on the commercial aspects of preventive medicine. They have, in particular, concentrated their efforts on screening programmes or medical checkups.

Checkups and screening examinations go back to the early part of the twentieth century. As long ago as 1917 more than ten per cent of the 300 largest American corporations were sponsoring regular examinations of their employees. When over half of 4 million draftees called up during the First World War were found to be either completely or partly unfit for military service American insurance companies became enthusiastic about the idea of screening the general population too.

(In the interests of historical accuracy I should perhaps mention that the first recorded 'screening' examinations were said to have been performed at a public brothel in Avignon in 1347. Every Saturday the women were examined by the Abbess and a surgeon. If they had caught any disease then they weren't allowed to work. But this was a very specialized form of screening.)

In Britain the screening-clinic boom has mostly been outside the NHS. Numerous commercial groups – some of them with powerful and rich American backing – have set up screening clinics where for a couple of hundred pounds it is possible to undergo a comprehensive medical checkup. Seeing the huge profits to be made by offering health checks, doctors within the NHS have desperately tried to climb aboard the bandwagon. The British Medical Association, the doctors' trade union, has argued that family doctors working within the NHS should be allowed to charge their patients up to £20 a time for routine health checkups.

For the private medicine industry screening is the biggest money-spinner since tonsillectomies went out of fashion. But despite the huge success of screening clinics, and the huge amounts of money being made by companies and doctors selling checkups to patients, there still isn't any evidence to show that screening does any good. Indeed, on the contrary, the available evidence suggests that screening probably does more harm than good.

As long ago as the early 1950s doctors were beginning to air their suspicions and fears about screening programmes. But it wasn't until more recently that hard evidence became available to show the uselessness of these examinations.

In the World Health Organization publication 'Measurement of Levels of Health' (published in 1979) there is a report entitled 'The Use of the Controlled Trial to Measure New Health Care Systems: Multiphasic Screening as an Adjunct to the United Kingdom National Health Service'. Two large group practices in South London were used for the experiment. All the patients in the two practices were aged between forty and sixty-four and were identified and divided into two groups. One group was the 'control' and the other group of patients was invited to attend a screening examination performed by nurses and supervised by a doctor.

This first examination was conducted in 1967 and three-quarters of the patients who were invited attended the screening examination. The patients had to answer a questionnaire, designed to find out if they had suffered any symptoms, they were interviewed, they were weighed and measured. They were given eye tests, hearing tests, chest X-rays, lung function tests, heart tests, and blood tests. Their blood pressures were taken, their faeces were tested, and they were given physical examinations too. They were, in short, given the sort of examination which in 1987 would cost approximately £200 when performed in a private clinic.

On average 2.3 diseases were found per person, although ninety-five per cent of the abnormalities were classified as minor. Many of the problems were already known about by the patients and their doctors but in all instances reports were made to the patients' GPs about any new findings. The first and most immediate problem discovered by the investigators was that in the vast majority of instances there was absolutely nothing they could do even when they had isolated and identified specific problems. 'Current medicine is limited,' they concluded, 'in its ability to influence the course of most chronic, degenerative diseases revealed by screening.'

The patients were invited back for further regular checkups during the seven years that followed. And at the end of the project – which lasted seven years and cost £275,000 a year – the health of the patients who had regular checkups was compared to that of the patients who had been the control.

The results were startling. Of the control group of 3,132 individuals 169 had died. But of the group who had been screened regularly 196 had died out of 3,292. There was no difference in the amount of sickness suffered by the two groups and the screened group had needed to go into hospital slightly more often than the control group. The results showed that if anything the control group was healthier.

As an incidental note it is perhaps worth recording that most of the doctors who helped with the screening found the work onerous and unrewarding. It was concluded that health screening is both expensive and ineffective.

The other major piece of medical research involving screening programmes was performed in Canada. The report of the Canadian Task Force on the Periodic Health Examination was published in the Canadian Medical Association Journal in 1979. The Task Force studied the question of medical screening for three years before coming to the conclusion that annual checkups should be abandoned since they were both inefficient and potentially harmful.

There are three main reasons why screening examinations are harmful. First, there is the problem that when people are taught to put their faith in medical checkups, they are encouraged to abandon any responsibility for their own health. If a patient goes to a screening clinic for a checkup and comes out with a clean bill of health, he is likely to leave quite happy that there is nothing at all for him to worry about. If he develops strange symptoms a week or a month later, he is likely to dismiss those symptoms as insignificant. He will have been misled into a false sense of security. Patients inevitably forget that a medical checkup is no more a sign of long-term health than an encouraging bank statement is a sign of permanent financial security.

The second reason why screening examinations are harmful is that they frighten people. In 1983 a psychiatrist at the University Hospital of South Manchester, Dr Peter Maguire, reported that since the start of screening in Manchester more women in their twenties and thirties had developed 'cancer phobia' while others had developed obsessional breast self-examination rituals. Other doctors have confirmed this danger. The main hazard seems to be that regular health overhauls which do not give the patient any real personal responsibility will lead to neurotic behaviour.

The third reason is that the procedures performed as part of a screening examination may do actual physical harm to a patient. There are, for example, some doctors who perform coronary angiographs as part of their checkup procedures. This diagnostic investigation involves pushing a catheter into the heart and then injecting a contrast medium and taking X-rays. There is a known mortality rate with this procedure. As many as one or two patients per 100 may die during the procedure.

And finally, of course, if a patient who has a checkup is then, as a result of the tests performed, subjected to other tests or to treatment which may not be necessary then his life will be threatened again.

Since the British and Canadian reports on screening many other surveys and commentaries have been published about screening. All the independent surveys and statements that I have found (the ones not made by people working for medical screening companies) have come to the same conclusion: screening is costly and useless. Even the President of the Royal College of General Practitioners, Dr John Horder, has confessed that health checks are a waste of time and money. It seems ironic that while the BMA has been campaigning for GPs to have the freedom to charge their own patients a fee for medical checkups, the RCGP should publish reports concluding that such checkups are not worthwhile.

CERVICAL SCREENING

Cervical-screening programmes regularly attract a considerable amount of publicity in the national press and in women's magazines. A number of extremely vocal campaigners have for some years now fought for more tests to be done and for more money to be devoted to cervical-cancer-screening programmes. Complaints commonly appear in the national press from observers who point out that there is no national policy on cervical screening and that while some women have annual smears other women have never had smears at all.

One gets the impression from all this publicity that many women now believe that if a properly organized cervical-smear programme were introduced, then thousands of women would be saved. This is simply not true. The fact is that cervical screening for cancer became established as a widely performed test long before any trials had been done to find out if the method was effective. No tests have ever been done to find out how best to use the technique and no attempts have been made to find out how to interpret the results. The chaos and confusion that exists in Britain at the moment is not a consequence of maladministration and incompetence; it is an inevitable consequence of ignorance.

The facts about cervical smears have been well documented in a number of scientific papers. One of the best and earliest review articles appeared in the *World Health Forum* in 1980. It was written by two women: Anne-Marie Foltz of the Graduate School of Public Administration at New York University and Jennifer L. Kelsey of the Department of Epidemiology and Public Health at Yale University.

Britain's cervical-smear programme is extremely expensive. It costs about £300,000 to identify every woman with cervical cancer and the screening system saves between five per cent and seven per cent of women suffering from the disease. I believe that if politicians, journalists and women's rights campaigners could be persuaded to study the evidence objectively, they would agree that the cancer-smear programme cannot be justified.

Here are the facts. First, although huge amounts of public money have been spent on organized cervical-screening programmes in recent years the incidence of cervical cancer has hardly altered in that time. After thirty years of cervical screening for carcinoma of the cervix, the incidence and mortality figures are falling, but the rate of decline is no greater than had already started before the cervical-screening programme began. Equally significantly, screening has also failed to produce a reduction in the incidence of the disease in many other countries. According to figures published in *Medical News* in July 1983 about 2,800 women died of cervical cancer in 1950. By 1966 the annual death rate from cervical cancer had fallen to 2,400. And by the early 1980s the cervical cancer death rate had fallen to around 2,000 – the figure at which it is still stuck. The fall in the number of women dying of cervical cancer has been steady but very slow. However, during the same period the number of cervical smears performed has rocketed. Back in 1966 about half a million smears were done every year. By 1982 three million smears were being done every year. We've been spending over £150 million a year on our cervical-screening programme since the early 1980s.

Second, although doctors have shown a considerable amount of enthusiasm for performing cervical smears they have never succeeded in deciding exactly which women need to be smeared. For many years now the system in Britain has been chaotic, expensive and ineffective. Women in one town are tested while women a few miles away are not tested. Some women under thirty-five have annual tests. Other, older, more-at-risk women have never had cervical smears done. The reason for all this confusion is that doctors still do not agree about when or how often smears need to be done to be useful.

It is, indeed, difficult not to be cynical about the enthusiasm shown by the medical profession. In one medical journal, *Financial Pulse*, recently a writer pointed out that 'unless doctors take urgent individual action a serious breakdown in cervical smear recalls – affecting GP income – could arise in five years' time'. From this it does seem possible that the chaos and confusion could be a result of the fact that the aims of those doctors performing profitable smears have been to maximize their incomes rather than to minimize the number of women suffering from the disease.

Third, cervical cancer is not as common a killer as many women believe. In Britain cervical cancer is responsible for 2,000 deaths a year, but far more women die of breast cancer, lung cancer, cancer of the colon, stomach cancer, and ovarian cancer. In 1985 the death rates respectively were 13,513; 9,798; 6,364; 4,049 and 3,843. Surprisingly cervical cancer does not figure in the top ten causes of death among women. Even carcinoma of the pancreas kills more women than carcinoma of the cervix. A modest expenditure on educational programmes could dramatically reduce the numbers dying of lung or breast cancer.

Foltz and Kelsey, in their article in *World Health Forum*, pointed out

171

that because the disease is relatively uncommon, huge numbers of women who do not have the disease are subjected to unnecessary tests and, because 'false positives' are fairly common, are referred unnecessarily for further tests and treatment. In my experience an enormous amount of anxiety and fear are produced by 'false positives' which are considerably more common than real 'positive' smears.

Fourth, and perhaps most significant of all, the smear test does not seem to be either accurate or reliable. Several surveys have shown that different cytologists reading the same slide report different results. Other surveys have shown that abnormal cells may be present in one sample and not in another from the same woman. Astonishingly, no proper tests have yet been done on the smear test. What is perfectly clear, however, is that many of the smears taken by doctors are useless. In an article in the journal *Modern Medicine* Dr Chandra Grubb, Director of the Department of Cytology at the Royal Free and University College Hospitals in London, has reported that an estimated ten per cent of all cervical smears sent to cytology departments are useless and that a further forty per cent are of limited usefulness in detecting carcinoma of the cervix. The main problems are that doctors either take smears from the wrong site or use faulty techniques.

Sadly, even when useful smears are taken the laboratories providing results cannot always cope. And even when laboratories do discover significant changes women aren't always notified.

In Oxfordshire in 1985 one woman who had had a positive smear test died before she was given her result. Another two became seriously ill. It turned out that doctors were not automatically telling women the results of their smears – but were waiting for them to make enquiries. Women who assumed that 'no news was good news' might as well have not had smears done at all.

The fifth problem is that there is still a considerable amount of confusion about the natural history of cervical cancer. From the evidence that is available it seems that some slow-growing cancers do regress if left alone while fast-growing cancers develop so rapidly that smears would have to be done every few months to be of real value. In the *Lancet* in 1978 Kinlen and Spriggs concluded that one-third of the biopsies, in which a small part of the cervix is removed, done in Britain because of positive cervical cytology are likely to have been performed for lesions which are insignificant or would have disappeared if left alone.

Since biopsies and other operations are performed under anaesthetic (with which there is always a risk of death) it seems perfectly possible that the dangers associated with having a smear done are greater than the possible advantages.

There is still a considerable amount of confusion among gynae-cologists about the best way to treat cervical cancer even when it has been identified.

With all this evidence available the conclusion has to be that the cervical-screening programme currently being run in Britain is expensive and worthless. As I have already pointed out elsewhere we can no longer afford to indulge our whims and spend huge sums of money on ineffective techniques.

But in view of the fact that many politicians, journalists, and women's rights campaigners have now convinced themselves that cervical screening is worthwhile it seems to me likely that the debate about which women should be screened, and how often they should be screened, will continue in Britain for many years to come. I doubt if anyone will have the courage to ask the as yet unasked question: 'Is cervical screening worth doing?'

I certainly doubt if doctors will ever want to hear that particular question asked. They, after all, have been making good money out of the cervical-screening programme for some years now. Neither GPs nor gynaecologists will want the system changed.

BREAST SCREENING

In February 1987 Norman Fowler, Secretary of State for Social Services, announced that the Government was setting up a national breast-cancer-screening service. Mr Fowler was, inevitably, bowing to a considerable amount of pressure from campaigners who had for several years been arguing that women should be given annual or six-monthly breast checks.

In a way it is more logical to spend money on a breast-screening programme than on a cervical-cancer-screening programme. After all, breast cancer kills far more women – around 13,500 a year – and, in addition, is responsible for a considerable amount of anxiety and distress. I suspect that breast cancer probably causes more fear and more loathing than any other type of cancer that exists. But is the Government's new breast-screening service going to make any difference? And is it going to be cost-effective? Or is it merely a sop to women politicians and journalists working for trendy newspapers and magazines?

Well, on the face of it the breast-screening programme certainly seems more sensible than the cervical-screening programme. The Government's plan is to screen all women between fifty and sixty-four once every three years and will use mammography – X-rays of the breasts – to enable doctors to make accurate diagnoses. However, one or two problems immediately need answering.

The Government's plan is to test only women between the ages of fifty and sixty-four but for women between the ages of thirty-five and fifty-four breast cancer is the commonest single cause of death. So, there will undoubtedly be a good deal of controversy about the proposed limits. Why should women under fifty be excluded from the screening programme? As long ago as 1981 there was an editorial in the *Journal of the American Medical Association* pointing out that if you're going to screen women for breast cancer, then you should screen all women over the age of forty.

The second problem is maintaining the quality of the screening service. If lots of false positives are found (in other words if lots of women who don't have breast cancer are told that they do have breast cancer), there will probably be a lot of healthy breasts removed from healthy women. As I have already pointed out (on page 67), there are still a good many surgeons in Britain who still believe that when a diagnosis of breast cancer is made then the breast should be removed.

The third problem is that screening women for breast cancer will be a labour-intensive activity. It will need a huge number of skilled doctors to do it properly. Way back in 1974 an editorial in the *British Medical Journal* pointed out that national breast-cancer screening would involve a third of all our surgeons doing nothing else all the time.

Now, one could argue that anything that kept so many surgeons out of the operating theatre would be a 'good thing' and that thousands of lives would probably be saved if the surgeons could be kept occupied in screening clinics. But the Government isn't going to use surgeons. It is going to use mammography (X-rays of the breasts) and the mammograms will be read by radiologists. That won't be a problem because by one of those wonderful coincidences it just so happens that for a while now Britain has been training thirty-two radiologists more than it needs every year. The new breast-screening programme will help mop up the glut of potentially unemployed radiologists.

But how good – and how safe – is mammography? It is difficult to say. Consultant Radiologist Dr Eric Roebuck told delegates at a Royal College of Radiologists' symposium early in 1987 that 'some existing centres are so bad – they have so many false positives and false negatives – that they positively do harm'. And there are, of course, risks involved in having regular X-ray examinations. No one knows just yet exactly what those risks are. We will probably find out in another ten or twenty years' time.

But these are largely hypothetical objections. My main objection to a mass breast-screening programme is simply that it won't work. It won't make a significant difference to the number of women dying of breast cancer because the interval of one year between examinations is too long.

If a woman has her annual screening test on 1 January and then develops a small lump on 1 February, it may well be eleven months before she sees her doctor again. She will be lulled into a false sense of security by the negative result of her January examination and she will be more likely to die of breast cancer than if she hadn't had the test.

I believe that the Government has only introduced breast-screening tests into the health service in order to satisfy the demands made by those who have allowed their emotions to overcome their judgement. For the plain truth is that it is far more effective, far more efficient, and far more economical to teach women how to examine their own breasts, at home, once a month. I make this claim not on subjective grounds but on the basis of sound scientific evidence.

In exactly the same month that the Secretary of State for Social Services announced that Britain would be offering a mammography service to a limited number of British women, medical journals were carrying firm evidence to show that home breast-testing really works.

Professor Martin Vessey and his colleagues in the department of community medicine and general practice in Oxford reported in the British Journal of Cancer that if women are taught how to examine themselves for breast lumps then cancerous lumps can be picked up at an early stage. Professor Roger Blamey, professor of surgical science at the City Hospital, Nottingham, and Jennifer Caseldine, superintendent radiographer at the Nottingham City Hospital's Helen Garrod breast screening unit, reported that after a six year study they had concluded that women who regularly examine themselves are able to detect cancers at a curable stage.

A proper educational programme, designed to teach British women how to examine their breasts properly, would undoubtedly have a dramatic effect on the number of women dying from breast cancer in Britain. It would cost very little and it would produce continuing results.

But it would not, of course, provide work for the thirty-two unwanted radiologists that we are training every year. And it probably wouldn't satisfy the strident spokeswomen who believe that annual screening clinics must be better than regular checks done at home.

175

SCANDAL No. 10

Ignoring the Power of the Mind

Less than ten years ago I wrote a book called Stress Control *in which I put forward the view that nearly all the common twentieth-century diseases are caused or made worse by stress. I argued that stress was the greatest environmental hazard of our time and that doctors should spend more time helping to manage stress, rather than merely treating symptoms.*

Many doctors with powerful academic positions laughed at the idea and dismissed it as fanciful nonsense. They still believed that all diseases had a physical basis. Today, most doctors admit that stress, fear, anxiety, worry, apprehension, anger, pressure, and even joy can all cause quite genuine physical responses and very real diseases.

But the majority of doctors are still reluctant to accept that although the mind can prove destructive, it can also have a remarkably powerful healing effect. Too many doctors still find the idea of patients 'thinking themselves well' or fighting disease with positive healing powers impossible to accept.

The majority of practising doctors are committed interventionists. They believe that when a patient is ill it is the doctor's job to make a diagnosis, to take charge, to provide a specific, prescribable treatment and to use physical forces to expedite a cure.

The figures vary from report to report but at a conservative estimate at least three-quarters of all the problems seen by doctors are illnesses which are either completely or partly psychosomatic in origin. If you include all the illnesses *not* seen by doctors – problems such as headaches, colds, mild anxiety, sleeplessness, back problems, period pains, and so on – then the figure will be even greater. I would estimate that between ninety and ninety-five per cent of all illnesses can be blamed totally or partially on psychological forces. Our minds are killing us.

Take the common or garden headache, for example. One of the commonest of all symptoms. There are some headaches that are caused by injury and a tiny number are caused by brain tumours but experts now agree that at least ninety-eight per cent of all headaches are stress- and pressure-related. When we are under stress we screw up our eyes, we tighten and tense the muscles around our heads – and we get headaches.

Some of the available evidence links stress to particular types of occupation. So, for example, the importance of industrial stress was first recognized in America in 1956 when a machine operator called James Carter cracked up while working on the General Motors' production line in Detroit.

Mr Carter had what is now commonly known as a nervous breakdown and he sued General Motors, claiming that the stresses of his job had contributed to his breakdown. It was an important lawsuit for Carter won and from that day onwards American industry took the relationship between stress and disease very seriously indeed. Since then researchers all around the world have published scientific papers linking specific occupations with specific types of stress-induced disease.

There have also been many papers published which have shown that social situations can cause damaging stress. In a paper presented to the American Psychiatric Association recently one author demonstrated that the immune system of a recently bereaved widow showed a marked reduction in efficiency – stress had changed her body's ability to cope with disease. Another report, this time published in the *Journal of the American Medical Association*, showed that the type of depression which is suffered following a bereavement can affect the body's internal defence mechanisms so violently that small, cancerous tumours which might otherwise have been suppressed by the body's own defences can survive, grow, and eventually kill the patient. A third study, this time published in Australia, showed that these changes in the body's internal immune responses and defences take place within a mere eight weeks of the death of a close relative. In other words, just two months after the death of someone close to us our bodies are so badly damaged by the stress that they become exceptionally vulnerable to cancers and infections of all kinds.

It isn't difficult to find practical evidence to support these studies. One partner dies and within a month or two the second partner, previously apparently fit and healthy, will die too. In one large study it was shown that the death rate among widowed individuals was twelve times the rate among a similar group of individuals who had not been bereaved.

There is similar evidence available showing that other social pressures cause problems too. If you are under pressure at home or your love life is too hectic, then your chances of having a heart attack are six times greater than normal. The same is true if you have money worries or problems involving close friends. If you are what is commonly known as 'socially mobile', then your chances of having a heart attack are increased by a factor of three or four.

Stress is, without a doubt, the major twentieth-century killer. But why? Why are we so much more susceptible to stress when, on the surface at least, our lives are so well organized? Most of us have enough to eat and somewhere to live. We don't have to worry too much about being eaten by wild animals. We have central heating and the choice of several channels of TV entertainment. Compared to our ancestors we have it easy. And yet we suffer more from stress than they ever did. Why?

The answer is simple: our bodies were not designed for the sort of world in which we live today. They were designed for a world in which fighting and running were useful practical solutions to everyday problems. Our bodies were designed for a world full of sabre-toothed tigers and physical danger.

Today we respond to threats in exactly the same way. When we have to face a problem our muscles tighten, our hearts beat faster, adrenalin surges through our arteries and our blood pressure goes up. We are physically prepared for action.

The trouble is, of course, that today's problems aren't quite as straightforward as yesterday's problems were. Instead of finding ourselves face to face with a man-eating sabre-toothed tiger, we are far more likely to find ourselves having to face unemployment, parking tickets, traffic jams, and gas bills. None of these modern problems can be dealt with by our physical responses, but we still respond in the same, old-fashioned way. We have not yet evolved enough to have 'learnt' that purely physical responses are no longer appropriate.

The real problem is, I suppose, that we have changed our world far faster than our bodies have been able to adapt. During the last couple of centuries revolutionary changes in medicine, printing, design, transport, agriculture, industrial methods, and communication systems have transformed our world. But our bodies are still much the same as they were 100,000 years ago.

When you're driving along the motorway and you see a police car in your mirror, your body will respond to the danger in the only way that it knows how: your heart will beat faster, your blood pressure will go up, your muscles will become tense, and your whole body will be prepared for a fight. Unfortunately, these simple physiological changes will not help you. Indeed, the responses are worse than useless. Your body will be frustrated because there will be no outlet for your physical responses.

Our world is full of problems which trigger off inappropriate physical responses. Pick up your morning post and find a rates bill hiding among the letters and you may well respond with tensed muscles, a faster heart beat, and raised blood pressure. These changes are quite inappropriate; they will not help you at all. But the changes take place because your body cannot differentiate between physical threats and financial threats. The damage that is done by twentieth-century stress is done through our minds.

And that leads me on to the next important part of this argument: it is not stress that does the damage; it is the way that we respond to stress. It isn't the rates bill or electricity bill that causes high blood pressure and ulcers; it is the way that we respond to the rates bill and the electricity bill.

Once again most doctors are now ready to accept this principle. During the last few decades a growing number of the world's 6,000 medical journals have carried reports providing evidence that illustrates the existence and importance of the link between mental responses and disease. In 1946, for example, a research project was started at Johns Hopkins University School of Medicine in Baltimore. The project involved nearly 1,500 medical students and was designed to investigate the relationship between attitudes and illness.

Seventeen years later the researchers came to the conclusion that the way an individual responds to pressure has a powerful effect on the types of illness that his or her body develops. It isn't just the stress that causes heart disease – it is the way that individuals respond to stress. This philosophy is explained in considerable detail in my book *Mindpower*.

The more researchers have investigated the power of the mind over the body the more they have become convinced that mental attitudes can even affect an individual's will to live. Most of us in the west think of voodoo as something of a joke. We think it slightly bizarre that there are still people living in Africa who can be so terrified by a threat uttered by a witch doctor that they will drop down dead within hours of being told that they are going to die.

But in essence we are no different. The only noticeable difference is that instead of wearing war paint, grass skirts and hideous masks our witch doctors tend to wear white coats and have stethoscopes hanging around their necks. When a doctor tells a patient that he or she has just three months to live then the chances are that the patient will duly die on time.

The only solid conclusion one can draw from all this evidence (and

179

there is a good deal more clinical and anecdotal evidence about the relationship between the mind and the body in my book *Mindpower*) is that the mind can have a very destructive effect on the body. Your mind can kill you, if you let it.

But there is another side to this argument; another aspect of the mind–body relationship that so far the majority of doctors have refused to accept. There is now a staggering amount of evidence to show that the power of the mind can have a remarkably constructive healing effect on the human body. The powers that can stimulate the development of disease can be used to stimulate the body's self-healing processes and to protect the individual from all sorts of diseases and disorders. The very same powers that can produce devastating damage can also be used to prevent illness developing and to deal with problems which have already started.

Although the clinical evidence supporting this philosophy has been slow to appear there have, in the last three or four years, been a whole host of papers published which have indicated that the healing power of the mind is far too important to be ignored.

One of the first experiments performed which showed the power of the mind took place in Australia in 1983. Researchers took a large group of people who had absolutely nothing in common apart from the fact that none of them had ever played basketball before. After being allowed to spend one day throwing basketballs through a hoop the volunteers were divided into three separate groups.

The first group was told to play absolutely no basketball for a month. They were told not even to think about basketball. The second group was told to practise every day. And the third group was told to spend ten minutes a day imagining that they were throwing balls into a basket.

At the end of the one-month experiment the people in the first group were no better at basketball than they had been at the start of the whole exercise. However, the other two groups had improved by closely similar amounts. The players who had been spending their time out on the court throwing basketballs through hoops had improved by twenty-four per cent. And the players who had spent ten minutes a day *imagining* that they had been throwing basketballs through hoops had improved by twenty-three per cent.

Numerous other sportsmen and women have confirmed the value of 'mindpower' in sport. In his book *Comeback: My Race For the America's Cup* yachtsman Dennis Conner wrote that: 'Another part of the psychological buildup had a lot to do with my theory that one's self image cannot distinguish between reality and a very vivid imagination. I tried to get the guys to imagine how good it would feel to execute the perfect cast-off or the perfect jibe. I asked them to imagine what it would be like to perform to complete perfection. I told them to capture the images of that perfection in their mind's eye. I asked them to use their affirmations to raise their self image in the same way that they used real life experiences to shape their own image of themselves. If you can visualize something, you can actualize it.'

Even more impressive has been the work done in America by Dr Carl Simonton and his wife. For a number of years now they have been teaching patients how to cope with cancer by using their imaginations. The theory is that if the imagination can have a destructive effect, it can also have a positive effect. If people can give themselves cancer by negative thinking, they should be able to protect themselves against cancer and maybe even cure themselves of cancer by positive thinking. In the first years of their experimental work the Simontons have found that their patients have lived, on average, more than a year longer than patients who were not encouraged to use their minds to help fight their disease.

All around the world doctors are now beginning to come up with similarly impressive results, often being able to show that the state of a patient's mind can have just as important an effect on his progress as the type of treatment he is offered. And there have even been papers showing that the attitude a doctor takes towards his patients will also have a powerful effect on the patient's chances of recovering.

So, for example, in May 1987 the *British Medical Journal* published a paper called 'General Practice Consultations: Is There Any Point in Being Positive?' The paper was written by Dr K. B. Thomas of the Department of Primary Medical Care at the University of Southampton.

For his research project Thomas took a group of 200 patients who arrived seeking advice from a GP. None of the patients had any abnormal physical signs and in none of the patients was any specific, definite diagnosis made.

The patients were then randomly selected for one of four different types of consultation. One group of patients were given treatment and also given what Thomas calls a consultation in a 'positive manner'. The second group were given no treatment but were given encouragement and given the 'positive manner' consultation. The third group were given treatment and a consultation in a 'negative manner'. The fourth group were given no treatment and no encouragement – they were given only a consultation in a 'negative manner'.

In 'positive manner' consultations the patient was told firmly that he would be better in a few days. In 'negative manner' consultations the patient was told 'I cannot be certain what is the matter with you'.

181

When treatment was given it consisted of a vitamin tablet prescribed as a placebo.

The results were very impressive. Thomas found that giving the patient treatment made little difference to the chances of the patient feeling better. But he did find that the patients who had had what he called a 'positive manner' consultation got better much quicker than the patients who had a 'negative manner' consultation. Two weeks after the consultation only thirty-nine per cent of the patients who had had the 'negative consultation' felt better whereas sixty-four per cent of the patients who had had the 'positive consultation' felt better.

I strongly suspect that in the next few years there will be many similar papers appearing in medical journals around the world. Doctors will be able to prove what has, in reality, been common knowledge for a long time: that the doctor who offers hope, reassurance and positive advice will have a much better healing rate than the cold, uncaring physician who relies entirely on pills. When a doctor gives a placebo it is not the pill that cures the patient's ailment; it is the encouragement and support that goes with the placebo. In short, it is the doctor who does the healing by introducing into the patient a feeling of confidence.

The scandal here is that the vast majority of doctors – at least ninety per cent – are still unaware of this 'mindpower' effect. They still practise in the old-fashioned, interventionist way and rely on pills and potions which have dangerous side effects when in reality they could get better results merely by changing their manner.

SCANDAL No. 11

Ignoring Social Factors in the Development of Illness

Most people who are ill do not need medicines. They don't need doctors, hospitals or drugs. They don't need scanners, coronary angiograms, electrocardiograms, electroencephalograms, barium-meal X-rays or intravenous pyelograms. They don't need transplant surgery, electroconvulsive therapy, corticosteroid drugs or benzodiazepine tranquillizers. They don't need physiotherapists, radiographers, chiropodists, osteopaths, acupuncturists, homoeopaths, hypnotherapists or chiropractors. They need a little more knowledge, a little more money and a little less worry.

In the last few years environmental experts have spent a lot of time and money investigating environmental pollution. They have studied at length the dangers associated with food additives, asbestos and radiation. They have, however, largely ignored the fact that ill health is far more commonly associated with social pressures such as unemployment, divorce, boredom, and frustration.

According to Professor Peter Townsend, of Bristol University, who is widely acknowledged to be one of Britain's leading experts on poverty, two-thirds of all serious health problems in Britain are caused by material deprivation. Chronic sickness, low birth weight, early deaths – all these are associated with poverty. Townsend claims that if saving lives is an important goal in Britain today then we 'must acknowledge that social policies to improve the worst housing and to improve working conditions are as necessary as good drugs'.

And all the historical evidence strongly supports his argument. There is now little disagreement among historians and statisticians that the massive improvement in health care that so marked the nineteenth century was a result not of better medical facilities, more doctors or more efficient drugs, but of better housing conditions, better working conditions, better roads, more food, cleaner water, and better sewage disposal facilities.

The nineteenth century saw many major medical advances including anaesthetics, asepsis, and widespread vaccination programmes. But these advances made very little difference to mortality and morbidity figures. The major advances were made through the efforts of social reformers not doctors.

But Townsend, and those who think like him, are not likely to find many supporters or sympathizers either within the medical profession or within the House of Commons. Doctors have a vested interest in campaigning for more money to be spent on health-care facilities. Their incomes and empires depend upon there being a strong and continuing support for orthodox ways of treating illness and combating death. Politicians prefer to side with doctors because they realize that genuine social reform is incredibly expensive and would be extremely unpopular with the wealthier citizens.

Indeed, some outside observers believe that it was the Health Education Council's attempts to publicize its own report identifying overcrowding, poor housing, and other economic problems as being largely responsible for the amount of ill health in Britain that encouraged the Government to shut down the HEC and replace it with the Health Education Authority (a body which is, I suspect, unlikely to risk upsetting anyone).

It seems unlikely that any real attempt will be made to improve the status of the millions whose lives are now deprived of hope or comfort. The divide between the two Britains seems certain to grow wider and wider during the next few years.

In the previous chapter I described how stress and pressure are common causes of illness. This is perhaps the time for me to crush a myth about stress that has now survived for far too long.

Mention the word 'stress' to most people and they think immediately of businessmen rushing from office to airport. The word 'stress' is usually associated with too much activity and too much responsibility. There is some truth in that association. People who push themselves too hard do suffer from stress-related disorders.

But the majority of people who suffer from stress aren't business executives rushing about from Geneva to Paris to New York to Tokyo. The majority of stress sufferers are people whose lives need more, not less, excitement.

Take stress among the employed, for example. In the previous chapter I mentioned the machine operator James Carter who is recognized as being the first employee to suffer from industrial stress. Carter wasn't an executive. He was a machine operator. And the chances are that his problems were produced not by excitement but by boredom and frustration. Stress on the factory floor or in the general office is a major but constantly unrecognized problem in Britain today.

I estimate that in 1988 stress will cost British industry something like £20,000 million. It will cost major companies about £1,000 for every employee. In an average lifetime the average employee will lose one and a half years from work because of stress-induced illness. Stress costs British industry at least ten times as much as strikes.

Certainly it is true that highly paid executives suffer from stress. But it is also true (and usually forgotten) that people working on the production line and in the accounts department also suffer from stress.

There are today millions of workers whose jobs demand that they act as nursemaids to expensive, complicated pieces of machinery which they do not understand. In factories there are pieces of machinery which can turn out an endless stream of finely finished objects. No craftsman working with his own hands could hope to emulate such accuracy. In offices there are computers and word processors which can write letters, check spelling, and keep files far more speedily and efficiently than any secretary could hope to do them. These days machines are so sophisticated that they are the principals in any working relationship. The individual is left little opportunity for pride or self-expression. Skilled workmen have no outlet for their skills. They are left frustrated and bored. Even brawn is out of style today. Today brawn and strength count for nothing. A wimp with a machine can do the work of ten strong men. Anger, frustration, despair, and violence are the inevitable consequence.

But it is perhaps among the unemployed, the great casualties of the Second Industrial Revolution, that stress wreaks most havoc. The unemployed have, by definition, little money. They tend to eat whatever is cheap (and that means whatever the food industry wants them to eat) rather than what is good for them. They are frequently cold and damp in the winter as energy bills rise. And they are shorn of all hope, ambition and self-respect.

For years now it has been widely acknowledged that there are many physical and mental problems known to be directly associated with unemployment. In Britain, as in many developed countries, there are now huge areas where unemployment hovers constantly between twenty-five and thirty per cent of the local workforce. According to American health statistician M. H. Brenner (American figures are easier to come by because in Britain information of this kind is usually suppressed by the Government) unemployment figures are the single most important economic index as far

185

as health is concerned. As unemployment rises so does alcoholism, heart disease, and admission to psychiatric hospitals. Studies have shown that unemployed workers are likely to suffer from indigestion, arthritis, high blood pressure, and a host of psychosomatic disorders. Brenner's figures show that when unemployment rises by one million in five years there will be 50,000 more deaths from general illness, 167,000 more deaths from cardiovascular conditions and 63,900 more admissions to psychiatric hospitals.

It has also been shown that disabilities or minor handicaps which did not prevent people from holding jobs deteriorated following a period of unemployment which could not be explained by the natural course of the illness. And there is also powerful evidence to show that an unemployed worker's family will also run a greater risk of falling ill. A major survey of unemployed families has shown that following unemployment children complained of gastrointestinal disturbances, suffered disturbances in eating and sleeping habits, and became accident-prone. Children were also more moody and developed behavioural disorders. A review of the relevant literature, written by Dr Leonard Fagin, appeared in *Update* in April 1983.

One of the few significant papers dealing with the relationship between unemployment and disease to have been published in Britain in recent years appeared in April 1987 in the *British Medical Journal*. Entitled 'Social Class, Non-employment, and Chronic Illness: Continuing the Inequalities in Health Debate' the paper was written by Sara Arber, Senior Lecturer in Sociology at the University of Surrey.

Arber confirmed that the lower-class unemployed people suffer far more ill health than unemployed people higher up the social ladder.

Earlier in 1987 the *British Medical Journal* published a paper entitled 'Unemployment and Mortality: Comparison of the 1971 and 1981 Longitudinal Study Census Samples.' This paper confirmed some of Brenner's American findings.

There can no longer be any doubt (if doubt there ever was) that poverty and unemployment are major causes of ill health in Britain. In an editorial published in the *British Medical Journal* in April 1987 the Assistant Editor, Dr Richard Smith, pointed out that 'it looks as if unemployment is still associated with a substantially increased mortality despite being a common experience' and he also warned that 'unemployment probably disables more often than it kills'.

SCANDAL No. 12

Problems with the Principle of Interventionism

The vast majority of orthodox doctors are committed interventionists. They treat their patients as battlegrounds, the illness as an enemy and their own armoury of drugs or techniques as weapons with which to fight illness.

The interventionist philosophy is so strong that many patients hesitate to deal even with mild symptoms without first asking for professional advice. The interventionists have gained total control of our health.

In many cases ignorance and fear combine to produce powerful and debilitating hypochondriasis. And yet calling in a professional is not always the right approach. The human body is equipped with an enormous range of subtle and sophisticated feedback mechanisms. The capacity of the human body to heal itself is far greater than many of us imagine.

Left to our own devices many of us could look after ourselves efficiently and safely.

We need doctors. We need doctors to look after broken limbs. We need doctors to remove ruptured appendices. We need doctors to prescribe antibiotics for pneumonia. We need doctors to treat a wide variety of specific medical problems. But in the last century or so doctors have taken on an increasing amount of responsibility for the health of their patients. Treatment has become doctor-orientated; patients have been encouraged to abandon themselves in the hands of their physicians. Instead of teaching us that our lives are in our hands doctors have taught us that our lives are in their hands. We have been taught to become dependent.

What doctors have not taught us – and what we have ourselves forgotten – is that the human body is well equipped to look after itself when threatened with disease and infection. The body's defence mechanisms and self-healing mechanisms are so effective that in at least ninety per cent of all illnesses patients can get better without any form of medical treatment. Among that ninety per cent of patients interventionism is only likely to lead to unnecessary side effects and unwanted problems.

Even the responses which seem relatively straightforward aren't always as simple as we imagine them to be. Our bodies are far more sophisticated than we expect. If you cut yourself, for example, you expect the blood to clot and the wound to heal. It doesn't seem like anything special or particularly complicated. In practice, however, the blood-clotting mechanism that you take for granted is part of a defence system that they would be proud to match in any science laboratory. A network of failsafe mechanisms ensures that the system isn't accidentally triggered into action when there is no leak. More safety checks ensure that the clotting system doesn't begin to operate until enough blood has flowed through the injury site to wash away any dirt which might be present. Once the clot has formed and the loss of blood has been stopped, the damaged cells will release into the tissues chemicals which are designed to make the local blood vessels expand. The expansion of the vessels ensures that extra quantities of blood flow into the injury site, the additional blood making the area red, swollen and hot. The heat will help damage any infective organisms and the swelling will ensure that the injured part is not used too much. By immobilizing the area the pain and the stiffness will act as a natural splint. White blood cells brought to the injury site help by swallowing up any debris or bacteria. These scavenging cells, bloated with rubbish, will allow themselves to be discharged from the body as pus once they have done their job. Then, once the debris has been cleared and the threat of infection removed the injury will begin to heal. The scar tissue that forms will be stronger than the original skin. All this assumes that the injury is a fairly small one and that the clotting mechanism can deal with the potential blood loss effectively.

If there is an appreciable blood loss, however, your body has a number of other mechanisms designed to help you stay alive. Arteries supplying the injured area will constrict so as to limit further blood losses. Peripheral blood vessels supplying the skin will shut down to ensure that the supply of blood to the more essential organs can be preserved. The kidneys will cut off the production of urine so that fluid levels within the body can be kept as high as possible. Fluids will be withdrawn from your tissues to dilate and increase the volume of the blood which remains. The red-cell-producing sites within your body will step up production in order to replace the cells which have been lost. Finally, as an added refinement, the loss of blood will trigger off a thirst intended to ensure that the missing fluids are replaced as soon as possible.

I have described the blood-clotting mechanism at some length not because it is particularly sophisticated or impressive, but because it is one of the *simplest* of all the body's defences! There are many more impressive defence systems.

Go out for the evening and drink several pints of fluid and your kidneys will get rid of the excess. On the other hand if you spend the day hiking in the sun, and you drink very little, your kidneys will reduce your fluid output. While they are regulating fluid flow your kidneys will also ensure that the salts, electrolytes and other essential chemicals in your body are kept balanced. Eat too much table salt, for example, and your kidneys will ensure that the excess is excreted.

There are mechanisms designed to keep your internal temperature stable. Sit in the sun and your skin will go pink as more fluid flows through the surface vessels of your body. This increase in superficial blood flow will enable your body to get rid of heat simply because the blood will lose heat to the surrounding air. You'll sweat, too, as your body cunningly uses the fact that, when water evaporates, heat is lost. As the sweat pours out, so the amount of saliva you produce will fall, thus making your mouth dry. You will get thirsty and drink more fluids to replace the fluid your body is losing.

Should a speck of dust find its way into one of your eyes, tears will flood out in an attempt to wash the irritant away. The tears contain a special bactericidal substance designed to kill off any infection. Your eyelids will temporarily go into spasm to protect your eyes from further damage.

When you have a fever, the rise in tissue temperature is probably a result of your body trying to help you cope more effectively with any infection that may be present. The temperature rise improves the capacity of the body's defence mechanisms while at the same time threatening the existence of the invading organisms.

And it seems, too, that there is sense in the old theory that it is better to starve a fever than to force food down an unwilling patient's throat. It seems that whereas the human body can survive without fresh food, living on its stored supplies, the bacteria which cause infection need fresh food if they are to live and breed.

Researchers have shown that the brain contains a natural form of Valium designed to help suppress anxiety; that pain thresholds and pain-tolerance levels increase quite naturally during the final days of pregnancy; that breast milk contains a substance designed to tell a baby when he has had enough to eat; and that during the years when a woman is fertile the walls of her vagina produce a special chemical designed to reduce the risk of any local infection developing.

Do a lot of kneeling on a hard surface and your kneecaps will acquire a soft, squashy, protective swelling. Eat something infected and you will vomit. Get something stuck in your windpipe and you will cough it up. Spend a lot of time in the sun and special pigmented cells will migrate to the surface of your skin to provide you with a layer of protection against the sun's rays.

The human body cannot always cope with disease itself, of course. There are times when even these immensely sophisticated self-healing mechanisms are overwhelmed and need support.

But to dismiss the effectiveness of these mechanisms and to deride the body's natural healing powers on the grounds that they don't always work is silly: it is like arguing that it isn't worthwhile learning to swim because occasionally you may need the help of a lifeguard. And yet that is just what doctors frequently do: they dismiss the body's healing powers as feeble and irrelevant. And they insist on intervening whenever infection or disease threatens.

What doctors tend to forget is that all symptoms are merely external signs that a fight is taking place inside the body. Unless the interventionist treatment is carefully designed to support and aid the fight, the treatment applied may well end up damaging and even weakening the body's internal mechanisms and eventually making the patient more vulnerable and more reliant on interventionists and their treatments. Twentieth-century interventionism is making us physically weaker.

We are less capable of coping with minor infections, minor anxieties and minor inflammatory problems because we have been treated with powerful drugs which have taken over from our natural healing mechanisms.

This problem is easily illustrated by referring to steroid drugs – extremely powerful products which mimic the action of the cortico-steroids produced naturally within the human body in response to threats of many different kinds. During the last few decades an increasing number of doctors have got into the habit of using artificial steroid drugs to treat problems such as arthritis and asthma. These drugs are powerful and effective and can suppress uncomfortable symptoms very quickly. But when a patient takes steroid drugs regularly his body's natural production of steroids falls. Eventually his body will not be able to respond to normal threats in the normal way. He will become dependent on artificial steroids. He will become exceptionally vulnerable to disease.

Twentieth-century interventionism is not only making us physi-cally weaker and more vulnerable. By making us more aware of our frailties and vulnerabilities and at the same time making us more dependent on health-care professionals (particularly doctors) the interventionists are turning us into a race of hypochondriacs. We are taught to fear disease but we are also taught to expect the professionals to look after us. We are repeatedly told that we live in a dangerous world but we are not told how to look after ourselves. We are told to be on the lookout for disease, but we are not told which symptoms are important and which can safely be ignored. This combination of fear and ignorance leads directly to hypochondriasis.

We are told to take more exercise. But we are told that exercise can kill. We are never told how much exercise we need and how much can prove fatal. We are told that coffee can cause cancer. We learn that tomatoes can cause cancer. We learn that animal fats cause heart disease. Then we read that fats are safe, that we should eat more tomatoes and that coffee is good for us. We are told that over-the-counter medicines are dangerous but the adverts tell us differently. We are told that we need vitamin supplements, iron supplements, zinc supplements, calcium supplements, and magnesium supplements. We are told to eat less salt but to eat more potassium. We are told to eat more fibre and to avoid overcooking our greens. We are told that too much vitamin C causes kidney stones. We are told to drink more milk. We are told to eat butter. We are told that milk causes heart disease. We are told that vitamin E can kill. We are told to take up aerobics. We are told that aerobics are dangerous. We are told to watch out for skin blemishes that change colour. We are told to keep out of the sun. We are told to get lots of fresh air. We are told to walk as much as we can. We are told to take up cycling. We are told to keep off the roads. We are told that we should take indigestion seriously. We are told to watch out for head pains because they can be a sign of developing tumours. We are told that breast lumps need identifying quickly. We are told that boredom kills millions. We are told that a low-fibre diet leads to bowel cancer.

It goes on and on and on. We are given thousands of conflicting warnings. We are given very little comfort, advice or encouragement to take responsibility for our own health. Is it any surprise that a recent survey showed that ninety-five per cent of the population say that they have had at least one bout of illness in any fourteen-day period?

SCANDAL No. 13

The Rise and Rise of Alternative Medicine

The popularity of alternative, or complementary, medicine has increased rapidly in the last few years. All around the world the number of people practising acupuncture, herbalism, hypnotherapy, and other forms of complementary medicine has increased annually. In just about every developed country in the world millions of people regularly seek help from alternative practitioners.

Many of the patients turning to these new branches of health care do so because they are dissatisfied with orthodox medicine. One hundred years ago people were so dissatisfied with orthodox medicine that they became Christian Scientists. Today patients turn to flower remedies or iridology. Patients are frightened by the high incidence of side effects known to be associated with modern drugs and surgical techniques, they are annoyed by the lack of time and courtesy offered by clinicians, and they are attracted by the promises and sympathetic manners of alternative practitioners.

But sadly many of the so-called 'experts' offering alternative advice are charlatans. Most are interventionists, following a philosophy as intrinsically old-fashioned and dangerous as orthodox medicine. Patients who, in good faith, seek honest advice and sympathetic support are too often likely to receive neither.

The boom years for alternative medicine have seen the development of a vast number of alternative specialities. Some such as homoeopathy are symptomatic. Some such as naturopathy are designed to improve the overall health of the individual. Some, such as biochemistry, are modern. Some, such as acupuncture, can trace their origins back thousands of years. Some, such as meditation, are based on unexplained mental powers. Some, such as reflexology, are based on physical philosophies. Some, such as herbalism, are clearly and unarguably interventionist. Some, such as massage, are logical and physical. Some, such as radionics and iridology, are irrational and illogical.

There has been an explosion in the number of practitioners

offering alternative-medicine services. Walk through any decent-sized town and you'll find rows of brass plates advertising the services of hypnotherapists, herbalists, and osteopaths. Let your fingers walk idly through the yellow pages and you'll find acupuncturists, homoeopaths, chiropractors, hydrotherapists, and a hundred and one other impressive-sounding specialists.

There are, surprisingly perhaps, no laws about who can or cannot practise alternative medicine. A man can leave his factory or office job on a Friday evening and set up shop as a hypnotherapist or herbalist on Monday morning. Many do. Nor are there any laws about who can or cannot offer diplomas or training to other would-be therapists. The man who sets up his surgery on a Monday morning can on Tuesday start his own training college and issue his own diplomas of proficiency.

Many of the most impressive-sounding diplomas and qualifications are meaningless. The letters that adorn the average practitioner's visiting card and brass plate refer to worthless qualifications that can, as often as not, be bought for a few pounds and a few hours superficial 'study'.

There are practitioners in all alternative medical specialities who know virtually nothing about anatomy or physiology. There are practitioners offering their services at highly inflated prices who couldn't pass a junior school biology examination.

In earlier chapters in this book I have pointed out that orthodox medical practitioners are often dangerous, inconsistent, badly trained, greedy, unscientific, and ignorant. All these criticisms are, I fear, also true of many who practise alternative medicine. Many of them excuse their ignorance or lack of training by claiming that the treatments they are offering are, at least, safe. This is simply not true. There are a number of very real dangers associated with all types of alternative medicine.

There is the very real risk that because of a poor training an alternative practitioner will make an incorrect diagnosis and treat a patient improperly. In one well-documented case a twenty-two-year-old woman died of tuberculosis after being treated with epsom salts, herbs, and a fruit diet by a homoeopath who thought that she was constipated.

There is the real risk that a treatment offered by an alternative practitioner will interact dangerously with a treatment offered simultaneously by an orthodox practitioner. Prescribed drugs and herbal products are, for example, particularly likely to produce a dangerous response. In theory patients should always tell their doctors when seeing alternative practitioners (and vice versa). In practice, however, many patients are too embarrassed to be honest and put themselves at risk by continuing with two different treatments at once.

And there are intrinsic dangers associated with alternative therapies even when they are practised competently. In January 1986 the *British Medical Journal* contained a report of several patients whose spinal cords had been damaged by osteopathic manipulation. Other reports have shown that there are real hazards with just about all alternative practices. The most hazardous speciality is probably herbalism.

On top of all these hazards there is also the fact that alternative medicine often does not work. Very few proper clinical trials have been done, but when trials have been organized the results have been disappointing. There are successes, of course, but these are often anecdotal or fortuitous.

Alternative practitioners brush aside failure by saying that the patient did not want to be healed, that the patient was contaminated by drugs or chemicals prescribed by orthodox practitioners, or by blaming some other outside force. The charlatan sells hope and comfort but often delivers very little in the way of real results.

And yet patients are often so full of despair and need that they struggle hard to convince themselves that the treatment they are using is working.

I remember once trying to convince a friend that her vitamin supplements were unnecessary. She insisted that she took them to stop her getting colds.

'But you've had three colds already, this winter!' I pointed out.

'I know,' she said. 'But think how many colds I'd have had if I hadn't been taking the vitamin tablets.'

HERBALISM

Herbalists claim, with some justification, that theirs is one of the oldest branches of medicine. They also claim that as practised today herbalism is one of the most powerful and effective of all alternative therapies. I have chosen it, therefore, to help illustrate this particular scandal.

There are 350,000 known species of plants altogether and about 10,000 of these have been tested for medicinal properties. There are some treatment guidelines available to herbalists but most practitioners seem to make up their own regimes. There is little continuity and apparently no logic to the type of treatment offered. The lack of consistency does, indeed, make herbalism look bizarre and rather unscientific.

For example, in one large book on herbalism I found a list of twenty-one different substances recommended for patients suffering from eczema. In another major herbal textbook there were eighteen remedies listed for the same condition. Only two of the plants on the second list appeared on the first list. Among the herbal remedies recommended for eczema I found: pansy compresses, carrot juice, watercress, spinach juice, comfrey poultices, great burdock tea, bergamot oil and strawberry-leaf tea. Many herbalists are not content to use just one product but will mix together a dozen or more different ingredients.

When I asked the major medical libraries to perform a search of the medical literature and look for papers dealing with herbalism I had very little success. Very few clinical trials have been organized to assess modern herbal products. One of the few properly organized trials concerned a herb called tripterygium wilfordii, which grows in southern China and which has, for centuries, been recommended as a treatment for joint pain. The Institute of Dermatology at the Chinese Academy of Medical Sciences extracted the active principle and found that it worked with moderate success. Unfortunately, like so many other products used for joint pains, the herb was found to produce a wide range of side effects including: gastro-intestinal disorders, skin rashes, period problems, sterility, and blood disorders.

I then looked at the dangers associated with herbal products. One of the main claims made by herbalists is that their methods are entirely safe. This simply isn't true.

Recently, for example, the *Adverse Drug Reaction Bulletin* (which does not carry any drug-company advertising) claimed that herbal remedies can be just as toxic as any other drugs and that their reputation for being safe was built back in the days when side effects weren't recognized or recorded.

There just isn't space here to list all the side effects of herbal products. But to illustrate my point I have picked out one or two of the commonest herbs and listed some of the side effects known to be associated with their use.

Comfrey: used in the treatment of wounds, fractures, ulcers and hernias, but can cause liver damage and may cause cancer.

Evening primrose: used for high blood pressure, eczema, multiple sclerosis and premenstrual tension, but can cause skin rashes, headaches, and nausea.

Feverfew: used to treat arthritis and migraine, but can cause mouth ulcers, abdominal pains, indigestion, and a sore tongue.

195

Ginseng: used as a sedative and an aphrodisiac and a tonic, but can cause high blood pressure, skin problems, breast pain, diarrhoea, and nervousness.

Hawthorn: used as a sedative and as a treatment for heart problems and menopausal problems, but it does have a powerful effect on the heart and its use needs to be monitored carefully.

Skullcap: used as a tonic, sedative and diuretic, but it can cause mental confusion, giddiness, and an erratic heart rate.

Valerian: used as a tranquillizer, but it can cause headaches, giddiness, spasms, excitability, and hallucinations.

Yarrow: used to treat high blood pressure, menstrual problems, colds, and fevers, but can cause skin problems, dizziness, and headaches.

Since herbalists often mix many herbs together the possible number of side effects that can be associated with a single treatment is enormous.

Finally, I should also mention that there is a risk that herbal products, far from being pure and natural, may become contaminated. In 1983, for example, the DHSS issued a warning about a kind of herbal tea made with comfrey leaves. Due to a mistake made in the packing process the leaves had been contaminated with belladonna (deadly nightshade) leaves. Obviously there were real risks for patients taking the product – a product which they probably assumed was entirely harmless. This type of hazard is particularly likely to occur when local herbalists try preparing their own products or when patients try treating themselves with herbs they have grown at home or picked from the hedgerows. But even when products are packed in commercial quantities and are not contaminated there are problems since it is difficult to judge the purity, quality and strength of an individual batch. Studies of ginseng, for example, have shown tremendous variations in quality. There are, it seems, seasonal variations in plants grown in different soils.

The real scandal here is not that there are so many people practising herbalism but there are no official controls on those who practise this or any other alternative medical speciality.

WHEN IS AN EXPERT NOT AN EXPERT?

Like most writers on medical topics I receive a constant supply of new books by alternative practitioners. Every day's post brings a new supply of books from writers promising new cures and new remedies. Many of the claims they make are absurd but their books sell because although we all want to be healthy, fit and slim most of us want to be healthy, fit and slim without having to make any real effort. We want to live to be 100 but we don't want to have to change our lifestyles. We want to avoid lung cancer but we don't want to have to give up smoking. We don't want to have heart attacks but we aren't prepared to give up butter. Health that comes in a gimmicky book is so much easier than health that has to be bought by learning a more sensible lifestyle.

But in addition to the more bizarre books, that make outrageous claims, there are some volumes which may to the uninitiated seem to offer extremely sensible, well-thought-out, well-documented, authoritative advice. I picked out two recently published books of this type. First, *The Natural Family Doctor* edited by Dr Andrew Stanway. Second, *Better Health Through Natural Healing* by Ross Trattler. I went through both books comparing the advice they offered. After all, if alternative medicine really is logical and sensible then there must be some continuity in what different authors recommend. I picked a handful of common symptoms at random and then checked through both books to see what recommendations they made. I haven't included all the recommended remedies here.

Measles: The Stanway book is quite dogmatic. For measles it recommends something called Euphrasia which sounds like an Egyptian princess but is apparently a homoeopathic remedy.

Trattler recommends tepid baths, hot baths, hot foot baths, hot ginger chest poultice, burdock, garlic, onion soup, pleurisy root, wild clover, yarrow, chamomile tea, sundew, and golden-seal tea. And a few other products too.

Varicose veins: The Stanway book recommends hamamelis, pulsatilla and vipera (all homoeopathic remedies), adding six drops of lemon oil to your bath and rubbing three drops of lemon oil on to the affected areas, making a cold compress with tincture of calendula and cold water, avoiding weight gain, taking regular brisk walks, wearing elasticated stockings and lying with your legs against the wall.

Trattler recommends vitamin A, vitamin B, folic acid, vitamin C, vitamin E, essential fatty acids, calcium, blackstrap molasses, bran, chlorophyll, garlic, lecithin, rutin, wheatgerm, and zinc.

If you followed the recommendations in just one of these books, you'd hardly have time to breathe. If you followed the recommendations in both books, you'd never have time to notice your varicose veins.

Cystitis: For the treatment of common or garden cystitis the Stanway book recommends no less than four homoeopathic remedies (cantharis, nux vomica, aconite, and dulcamara). You choose your remedy according to your type of cystitis. So, if you think you got your symptoms after getting chilled in cold weather you take aconite. If you got your symptoms after getting chilled in cold wet weather you use dulcamara. The Stanway book also recommends that readers consult a medical herbalist for a diuretic herb. And it recommends cutting out meat, eggs, and citrus fruits, fasting for forty-eight hours and following a raw food or light diet. Finally it recommends taking contrast sitz baths daily, in which part of your body is immersed in cold water and part in warm.

Trattler recommends vitamin A, vitamin C, folic acid, pantothenic acid, niacin, vitamin E, acidophilus, chlorophyll, garlic, bearberry, buchu, comfrey, couch grass, goldenseal, juniper berries, marshmallow root and parsley root, and seed. It also suggests potassium broth, parsley tea, watermelon seed tea, cranberry juice, asparagus, parsnips, hot compress, and hot sitz baths.

Sadly the type of sitz bath varies. Stanway recommends filling one large bowl with cold water and another with hot. You sit in the hot bowl with your feet in the cold bowl for three minutes. You then reverse your position for one minute, and repeat this at undefined intervals.

Trattler recommends sitting in a container which is filled with hot water. He suggests that you do this for between three and ten minutes. He adds that you may rub yourself with a loofah mitten occasionally.

At first, when I saw the huge list of possible remedies I was amused. When I realized that nothing on one author's list appeared on the other author's list I imagined that most readers would find the advice farcical. Then, when I realized that *real* patients with *real* ailments and *real* fears will probably read no more than one of these books and try to deal with their problems according to the advice it contains I became angry.

It is, I believe, a scandal that authors and publishers should be allowed to continue selling advice of such doubtful value.

SCANDAL No. 14

Rapidly Changing Demographics

In the next fifty years age will probably have a far more divisive effect on our society than sex, race or class have ever had.

In the decade between 1971 and 1981 the total population of Britain increased by less than one per cent while the pensionable population rose by ten per cent. One person in five in Britain is already a pensioner and the proportion of people in their seventies and eighties is increasing rapidly too. By the year 2020 a third of the British population will be of pensionable age.

Those millions will need care, attention, time and money. But who will provide what they need? The scandal is that neither the medical profession nor the politicians have planned for the future.

People may not be healthier than they were. Thousands may be dying in their thirties and forties. Suicide and heart disease may claim the lives of many young adults still in the prime of their lives. But the size of our ageing population is expanding rapidly. The 1981 census showed that there were 6,500,000 women in Britain over the age of sixty. It showed that there were 3,200,000 men over the age of sixty-five. One-third of all adults in the United Kingdom is now over the age of fifty-five. The number of people over sixty-five in Britain has doubled in the last twenty years. Mortality among thirty- and forty-year-olds may have increased but the size of our pensionable population is expanding rapidly.

Much the same is true of other countries. In Sweden it has been estimated that between 1980 and 1990 the number of people alive in their eighties and nineties will double. (That means that the children of these elderly people will also be of pensionable age – there will be two generations of the same family requiring care and attention at the same time.)

By 2020, according to a recent study for the International Monetary Fund, nearly twenty per cent of the population of the seven most prosperous countries will be aged sixty-five or over. In West Germany and Japan, by 2020, one person in ten will be seventy-five or more. A massive forty per cent of West Germany's adult population of working age will be fifty or more.

Inevitably, much the same sort of thing is happening in America, too, where any rise in life expectancy is almost entirely due to a decline in the death rates among those aged sixty-five and over. There are, today, literally hundreds of thousands of Americans living well into their seventies, eighties and nineties. Eileen Crimmins, a researcher at the University of South California's Andrus Gerontology Center has forecast that if current trends continue life expectancy could increase by another twenty to thirty per cent by the early part of the twenty-first century – entirely as a result of the increase in the number of people surviving into their eighth, ninth, and tenth decade.

Several things make this explosion in the size of the elderly population particularly dangerous. First, there is the fact that among older populations there is inevitably a higher proportion of disabled and dependent individuals. I'm not just talking about the natural frailty that accompanies old age but about the fact that the incidence of chronic disease rises rapidly among older age groups. Among sixteen- to forty-four-year-olds twenty per cent of the population suffer from chronic illness. Among forty-five- to sixty-four-year-olds forty per cent of the population suffer from chronic illness. Among sixty-five- to seventy-four-year-olds fifty per cent of the population suffer from chronic illness. And among people aged seventy-five or over sixty-five per cent will suffer from chronic, long-term illness.

The size of the potential problem can be gauged from the fact that thirty-four per cent of the population already have poor health, affecting their ability to look after themselves. Writing in the *British Medical Journal* in January 1987, Robert Anderson, Senior Research Officer at the Institute for Social Studies in Medical Care in London, estimated that there are already more than 1,250,000 people in Britain caring for disabled or elderly people living in the community.

To illustrate the sort of impact this increase in illness is likely to have, consider blindness – just one of many chronic problems. Among the populations of most developed countries the incidence of blindness runs at about 200 per 100,000 people. But the incidence of blindness increases rapidly among older sections of the community. There are, for example, an average of 2,300 blind people out of every 100,000 citizens over sixty-five. Among over seventy-fives the incidence of blindness rises to just under 8,000 per 100,000.

Or consider strokes. Already half the beds in NHS hospitals are occupied by patients suffering from some form of stroke. Stroke patients generally need to stay in hospital for long periods of time and they need intensive nursing and medical care.

Or consider diabetes – a disease where the picture is rather more complicated.

A little over half a century ago diabetes was a killer disease. There was no available treatment. And so people acquiring the disease died at an early age. It was a fairly rare disorder. And then in 1921 Banting, Best and Macleod discovered insulin.

The effect was dramatic. Thousands of diabetes sufferers who would have died without insulin were able to live, marry and have families of their own. But since diabetes is a hereditary disease this inevitably meant that the incidence of diabetes in society increased at a rapid rate. By 1984 it was reliably estimated that one in every fifty people living in a developed country was a diabetic. Moreover, experts estimated that the incidence of diabetes is now doubling every decade and that although dietary habits may be partly responsible for the increasing incidence of the disease the genetic factor is the most important one. (Reports suggesting that the incidence of diabetes is doubling have come from several countries. In an article published in the *British Medical Journal* in 1983 Drs Stewart-Brown, Haslum and Butler from Bristol pointed out that 0.01 per cent of children born in 1946 had developed diabetes by the age of eleven; that 0.06 per cent of children born in 1958 had diabetes by the age of eleven and that 0.13 per cent of children born in 1970 had diabetes by their tenth birthday. Child-onset diabetes is usually more serious and difficult to treat than the more common adult-onset diabetes – which is also increasing rapidly.)

If the experts are right – and there is no reason to think that they aren't – then by 1994 four per cent of the population of Britain will be diabetic. By 2004 eight per cent of the population will be diabetic. By 2014 sixteen per cent of the population will be diabetic. And by the year 2020 nearly one in every four people will be diabetic.

It will be the genetic factor which will be primarily responsible. But it will have been our ability to keep diabetics alive into their seventies and beyond which will have turned a theoretical problem into a practical one.

Among the genetically transmitted diseases it is not, of course, simply diabetes which is increasing at such a rate. Among the many other genetically transmitted physical diseases which are increasing rapidly throughout the developed world are heart disease, strokes, congenital malformations of many different kinds and asthma. As with diabetes the basic explanation is simple. Fifty years ago a child with a congenitally deformed heart would have died. Today surgeons can perform repair operations that will enable that child to live to adulthood and to have children of his or her own. The incidence of that disorder increases with each new generation.

Nor is this developing problem confined to physical disease. There is ample evidence to show that mental disease is on the increase too. In the decade between 1973 and 1983 the number of patients with mental illness needing to be admitted to hospital rose by nearly ten per cent. Today in developed countries around the world it is widely recognized that between ten and fifteen per cent of the population will, at some stage in their lives, suffer from mental illness severe enough to warrant their admission to a mental hospital. Once again, the increase in the size of our elderly population is at least partly responsible for this increase in the number of mentally ill or disturbed patients in our community.

As the number of disabled older people increases, so more acute hospital beds will be blocked and unavailable for emergencies. Dr John A. Loraine, Senior Lecturer in the Department of Community Medicine and Director of the Centre for Human Ecology at the University of Edinburgh, has estimated that by 1992 ninety-four per cent of all non-maternity beds for women and seventy-five per cent of all beds for men in non-psychiatric hospitals could be filled by patients aged sixty-five or over.

Some experts would probably argue that blocking our hospital beds in this way will reduce the incidence of iatrogenic disease. But it will also increase the number of people in our community who suffer from disabling problems (such as arthritic hips) which could otherwise have received treatment. The inevitable consequence of that will be that the size of our disabled population will grow even faster.

To all this we must also add the fact that in Britain the average cost of health care for individuals aged between sixty-five and seventy-four is two and a half times as much as it is for those individuals aged between fifteen and sixty-four. For individuals over the age of seventy-five the cost of providing health care rises to seven times the cost of looking after patients who are under sixty-four. So, this steady increase in the size of our aged population will also ensure that the NHS will become increasingly short of funds.

The second factor which makes this explosion in the number of elderly people even more significant is that while the number of old people in our society is growing the number of young people is falling.

There are several reasons for this. The main reason is that while doctors have been extremely efficient at keeping elderly patients alive they have also been extremely successful at teaching younger patients to practise birth control. And so while the number of over sixties continues to increase rapidly the number of children growing up in developed countries is falling. Citizens in developed countries around the world have responded responsibly to an awareness of the world's overpopulation problem. The end result will be that by the time the 'baby boomer' generation has reached retirement age the number of healthy young and middle-aged adults able to work and care for the elderly population will, in proportion, be even smaller. In France some pressure groups, already aware of this potential problem, are enthusiastically encouraging young parents to have as many children as they can possibly afford.

The fall in the number of babies born during the 1960s, 1970s and 1980s is the main reason why the size of tomorrow's healthy young adult population will be far too small. But it isn't the only reason.

Another problem is that while people in their sixties, seventies and eighties are now living longer and longer, death rates among people in their twenties and thirties seem to be increasing. For example, the number of young people (particularly men) dying of heart disease is still rising in Britain. Less significant in numerical terms is the fact that the number of young people committing suicide is rising at a terrifying rate (see page 92). The result is that the imbalance between the size of our healthy young adult population and the size of our disabled and dependent elderly population will become even more dramatic. A smaller and smaller working population will have to support a larger and larger dependent population.

The third reason why the explosion in the size of the over-sixty population is likely to produce problems is financial.

In Britain – as elsewhere in the developed world – workers who are currently paying pension contributions assume that the money they are paying will be invested and repaid to them when they reach pensionable age. That is not the case. The state pension contributions paid by today's workers are used to pay the pensions of yesterday's workers – today's pensioners. The state pensions that today's workers will receive when they retire will be paid by the regular contributions made by tomorrow's workers. It doesn't take much imagination to see the sort of problems that are likely to arise.

The welfare state, originally designed to save society, may well turn out to be its ruin. Welfarism started to outgrow good sense in the 1960s. Like a baby cuckoo overtaking its putative parents Britain's welfare policies began to grow at an outrageous and unsupportable speed. An expanding economy and a massive influx of North Sea oil money partly provided the Government with increasing tax revenues and made it easy for it to gain political approval (and win electoral support) by pouring billions into welfare arrangements.

Today, however, the administration of social policies has put a huge administrative and tax burden on our society. At the moment thirty per cent of all public expenditure is on social security. One-third of the money we spend as a nation is pumped into the welfare state. A growing proportion of that money goes into looking after the ever-expanding population of pensioners.

This hasn't only happened in Britain, of course. During the 1970s and early 1980s the number of people in other developed countries receiving pensions, disability payments or other government support has risen rapidly.

For example, in 1968 in the Netherlands 5.5 per cent of the workforce were receiving disability benefits. By 1980 thirteen per cent of the workforce were receiving disability benefits and a similar number were receiving temporary sickness benefits. Today welfare costs amount to thirty per cent of the country's annual budget of $150 billion and the Dutch need a two per cent increase in annual production simply to maintain benefit payments at their present level.

In France social security and medical costs rose from $31 billion a year in the early 1970s to $124 billion a year in the early 1980s. In Sweden one-quarter of the country's economic growth is required simply to keep pensions in line with inflation.

All around Europe the number of individuals dependent on governments for their income has risen dramatically. As the number of people receiving public benefits has risen so the number of public employees hired to dispense those payments has also increased. The key years were the 1970s. Between 1974 and 1979 the number of people in Denmark working for private employers fell from 420,000 to 380,000 while during the same period the number of people working for the government rose from 550,000 to 750,000. In 1986 in Britain one-half of all adults depended on the government for their income – either because they receive public benefits (pensions, sick pay, and so on) or because they work as civil servants. For twenty years now in Britain as in most European countries only the public sector has created new jobs. Not even denationalization has halted the trend. Because of the demands of welfarism there has been no capital available to create new jobs or new real income. Fat cat civil servants, protected by index-linked pensions, have acquired all the authority while the responsibility for providing an ever-increasing standard of living has remained with those in the private sector. The welfare system has become so incomprehensible that not even experts working within it understand it properly. The system invites abuse and false claims.

As our frail, ageing, dependent, disabled population increases so the problem will continue to get worse. Already dissent and dissatisfaction are brewing. Taxpayers already feel aggrieved at the fact that they have to support the unemployed, the disabled, and the elderly. Things aren't helped by the fact that some of today's pensioners are better off than the people who are working to support them. In Britain the disposable income of the average pensioner has risen from about forty per cent of that of non-pensioners in 1951 to nearly seventy per cent today – and the expenses of pensioners are often much lower (there is no mortgage to pay, no children to look after, no work clothes to buy, and no travelling expenses to and from work – in addition pensioners usually get subsidized public transport and subsidized entry to cinemas, etc.).

By the year 2000 an even greater percentage of pensioners will have an overall income matching or exceeding the incomes of those who are working to support them. What will happen when the number of pensioners exceeds the number of workers – as it will early in the twenty-first century?

So far I have mentioned only the problems faced by the Government and I have referred only to state-paid pensions. But companies are going to face the same problems too.

An article in *Fortune* magazine in March 1987 spelt out the problems. The title of the article was 'Sick Retirees Could Kill Your Company' and the author pointed out that in 1974 the average Fortune 500 company (the 500 biggest companies in America) had twelve active employees for every pensioner. 'Today,' the author added, 'the average company has three active employees for every pensioner.'

In some firms the situation is already far worse. One large steel company had 70,000 workers and 54,000 pensioners just five years ago. Today that same steel company has 37,500 workers and 70,000 pensioners. In 1985 alone General Motors spent $837 million on the medical bills of its 285,000 pensioners and their dependents.

The situation is already desperate. It can and will get worse. As the number of seventy-, eighty- and ninety-year-olds in our society increases so the pressure on the remaining thirty-, forty- and fifty-year-olds will increase. As the number of people needing full-time medical care increases so the NHS will find it more and more impossible to cope.

It is salutary, perhaps, to remember that in Oxford the Regional Health Authority has already suggested that the only way it can possibly manage to maintain essential, basic services for its elderly population will be to withdraw the sort of comprehensive health care normally associated with the NHS.

I suspect that by the time we reach the end of the century the size of

Britain's elderly population will have begun to concern every politician, every doctor, and every administrator working within the NHS. By then it will be far too late.

EPILOGUE

Consequences

If none of the scandals I have described is opposed or controlled, the consequences will be horrendous. It could break down society completely.

Members of the shrinking able-bodied, employed community will rebel against the enormous burden they are forced to carry. There will be a growth in the black 'cash' economy. More and more people will voluntarily choose not to work but to accept social-security payments. The number of people working in productive jobs will shrink. And the pressure on the remaining workers will become intolerable. They will either abandon their burdens or they will demand enormous financial compensation. Inflation will become rife. The rift between the two Britains – the north and the south, the unemployed and the employed – will become wider and wider. The split between the 'haves' and the 'have nots' will reach new levels of unacceptability.

There will be a resurgence of Luddism with angry mobs smashing computers. And there will be a sharper than ever rift between those who receive social-security payments and those who hand them out. Men and women on both sides of the counter will be angry and bitter.

Taxes will rise to unacceptable levels. The social and medical services will break down completely. The western civilization that we know could collapse far more speedily and dramatically than the Roman Empire fell over a thousand years ago. No 'developed' country will escape the consequences, but it will be in Britain, where welfarism has reached a peak, that the problems will be at their worst.

There will be anger, frustration and bitterness. Society will break down into many different factions. There will be a rift between those who are public employees and those who are private employees – the former having total job security and the latter having no such security. There will be a rift between the young and the old with the old demanding better pensions and, by virtue of their very numbers, having enough political clout to ensure that they get exactly what they want. In a country where anything up to half the electorate are receiving pensions the political clout of the retired will be enormous. And in 2020 the eighty-year-olds will be members of the rock'n'roll generation – vocal and forceful. As the young see the elderly living better and better they will find their own falling standards of living unacceptable.

I fear that the rift between the able-bodied and the disabled will widen too. There will be resentment and bitterness and the shrinking able-bodied community will speak out openly against the disabled, the frail and the elderly. Hidden, unspoken fears will explode into the open. The able-bodied will complain about having to pay for the disabled. The employed will object to supporting the unemployed. The elderly will push aside the handicapped in the shops.

The result of all this will be that the moral climate of the country will change. People will demand action that we today would consider barbaric. There will be protests about hospital beds being blocked by the elderly, and chronically sick. There will be anger about the expenditure of money on performing surgery to save the congenitally deformed or the seriously injured. There will be calls for euthanasia to be legalized. Acceptable, humane manslaughter will be a legal defence in 'murder' cases. Unacceptable solutions will suddenly not only become acceptable but will become essential. Medical help will be available only to those who have power or who can show that they deserve it. Smokers will be denied medical help when they get bronchitis. Drinkers will have to accept death when they develop liver diseases. Political extremists will call for breeding licences for humans. Would-be parents carrying genetic traits of diseases such as diabetes will not be allowed to have children.

You may scoff and say that none of this could happen in our society. But it is already happening.

Drug addicts don't always get proper medical help. Smokers have been turned away by doctors and hospitals. Kidney transplants are performed only on patients with jobs, families and prospects. More and more people are calling for euthanasia to be legalized and legitimized. There is already a lack of compassion for the elderly, the disabled and the sick. And there is growing resentment against those who rely on social security benefits of any kind.

In one generation we have turned our society upside-down. We have gone from a baby boom to a situation where the fastest growing segment of the population is people over the age of seventy-five. The modern miracle technologies keep sicker and sicker patients alive longer and longer. Medicine has lost touch with reality; doctors have lost touch with patients. Aims and ambitions are distorted and confused.

I believe that the evidence shows that by the time we reach the year 2020 it will be too late to do anything to prevent the holocaust. Our society will be so weakened and so divided that recovery will be impossible.

In Britain one-third of the population will have reached retirement age. And at least one-half of the remaining adults will be chronic invalids, requiring permanent care and attention. Every single healthy adult in Britain – and elsewhere in the developed world – will be working to support three people and will have the physical responsibility of caring for three people too.

The year 2020 is significant because I estimate that that is the year when the number of disabled and dependent individuals in Britain will exceed the number of able-bodied individuals. And if that sounds unlikely then let me just remind you that today, on average, one-third of the population of any developed country will have such poor health that their ability to work or look after themselves will be seriously affected.

In the past threats to the survival of the human race have always come from outside. We have been threatened by infectious diseases. Or by starvation due to failing crops. Always we have been threatened by problems which we could counteract by trusting our scientists to work together and come up with a solution.

When we were threatened with starvation our scientists found new ways of harvesting food. And to protect us from future problems they developed better agricultural techniques. When we were threatened by infection our scientists developed better water supplies, better sewage disposal, quarantine, vaccination, and antibiotics.

This time the difference is that it is our scientists who have helped to produce the problems we face. The aims and aspirations of medical scientists once dedicated to eradicating disease have been distorted by professional ambitions and commercial forces.

In the past the most powerful forces in our society have always combined to oppose any threats from outside. Today the most powerful forces in our society – science and commerce – are conspiring to make things worse. The very people whom we might expect to help us deal with our problems have (perhaps because they don't understand what is happening) dedicated their lives to making the problems worse. Our medical scientists are so preoccupied with finding solutions to today's immediate problems that they have failed to understand the enormity of the dilemma in front of us. And the most powerful forces in commerce are so preoccupied with making profits for today that they have failed to see that they are helping to ensure their own eventual destruction.

If we do not take drastic action now, then all the evidence suggests that within our lifetime civilization will end. Forever.

For the first time in history the size of the population needing care and attention will exceed the size of the population fit enough to do the work and do the looking after. And the situation will then rapidly get worse and worse as each month passes.

Genetic influences will ensure that diseases become more and more common. The majority of the population will be disabled by disorders such as diabetes, epilepsy, heart disease, arthritis and schizophrenia. We will have defied nature and ensured the survival of the sickest.

The pressure on the healthy individuals who remain will be tremendous. Hospitals and nursing homes will be quite unable to cope with the demands for full time nursing care. In a household consisting of two healthy parents and two healthy children there will be at least four physically dependent relatives.

Ghettoes will spring up where the disabled and the chronically sick will be left to care for themselves and for one another.

But there are things which we can do now, and in the next decade, which will postpone the point at which the worst will happen and therefore give us a chance to find a more permanent solution to the problems I have outlined. But there isn't a day to waste. We must take action now if we want to avoid the holocaust.

CONTROLLING OUR DESTINY

A study of the scandals outlined in this book will have given you a very good idea of the changes we must make in our society if we are to survive. But on the following pages I have outlined some of the specific actions I believe we should now take if we are to approach the year 2020 with confidence and hope.

PREVENTIVE MEDICINE

More than fifty per cent of premature deaths are due to unhealthy behaviour and lifestyle while another twenty per cent of premature deaths are the result of environmental factors. Environment and lifestyle are far more important than medical services. Doctors should stop treating people just when they are ill and start treating them when they are well. No amount of medical attention can do a cigarette smoker as much good as teaching him how to stop smoking.

Sadly, at the moment, the NHS is sickness-orientated rather than health-orientated. At least ninety-five per cent of the NHS budget is spent on treating sickness rather than promoting or maintaining good health. Doctoring has become merely the art of curing illness; it has become divorced from people and science and has become merely a minor branch of twentieth-century technology. If we are to avoid the horrors of 2020, then the medical profession must change its policy from curative medicine to preventive medicine.

It is not difficult to see why the medical profession directs most of its attention towards curing existing illness. Traditionally, doctors have always been paid for providing treatment – whether pills or surgery – and the result is that there is today a huge 'industry' which has a vested interest in maintaining the status quo.

During recent years the medical profession has expanded at such a rate that there are today far too many physicians and surgeons and hospital beds in Britain (see p. 126). The amount of money spent on organized, orthodox health care is absurd. Patients have been encouraged to hand over responsibility for their own health with disastrous results. There are now millions of patients who will not deal with any problem – any minor illness – without first obtaining professional advice. Expectations have been raised to unreasonable levels. Millions of patients have been misled by the medical profession and expect an unreasonable quality of medical care. To all this we must add the fact that there is now an epidemic of iatrogenic illness. In 1973 doctors in Israel went on strike for a month. The death rate for the country dropped by fifty per cent – the largest decrease since the previous doctors' strike twenty years earlier! In 1976 doctors in Bogota, Colombia went on strike for fifty-two days with a thirty-five per cent fall in the mortality rate. Also in 1976 a doctors' strike in Los Angeles produced an eighteen per cent reduction in the death rate. During the strike there were sixty per cent fewer operations in seventeen major hospitals. After the strike was over, the death rate returned to normal.

But doctors don't just kill people. They also make people ill. People are not living healthier lives. It isn't the mortality rate that is threatening us. It is the morbidity rate.

One vital solution is for doctors to take preventive medicine more seriously. Instead of being a medical 'backwater' preventive medicine has to become the main firing force of the medical profession. We need constantly to remind ourselves that the main advances that have been made in medicine in the last century have been made not by individual surgeons or physicians performing operations or doling out pills, but by men and women who have taken a real and enthusiastic interest in keeping people healthy rather than treating them when they fall ill. Medical historians are now agreed that the most dramatic improvements in life expectancy were made long before the discovery of asepsis, anaesthesia or antibiotics. The nineteenth-century medical men who gave us better health and longer lives were the reformers who helped install better sewage facilities, provide cleaner water supplies and better housing.

We need to attack medical problems in a similar way today. The evidence shows that the vast majority of diseases can be prevented. We need new aggression and a new sense of urgency. And we need to give those who practice preventive medicine more political muscle.

Tackling health problems in this way will give us another advantage too. A traditional, interventionist approach inevitably increases the size of the disabled population – and puts additional strain on the welfare system. An approach designed to help keep people healthy reduces the strain on the welfare system and helps to produce a fitter population.

RESEARCH

We need to halt all medical research programmes immediately. Medical research programmes are invariably designed to search for new 'cures', new ways of keeping people alive and new ways of combating existing disease. These research programmes are inappropriate for several reasons.

First, we already have far more information than we can possibly use. Back in 1974 Professor Jean Hamburger, Professor of Nephrology at the Faculty of Medicine in Paris, wrote that 'even in a speciality as narrow as transplant immunology my laboratory has to subscribe to thirty-one different journals from which in one year alone we extract, catalogue and file over 5,000 articles. In short even the specialist is unable to keep pace with the growing mass of new data.'

Elsewhere it has been estimated that twenty per cent of all research work is unintentionally duplicated because research workers in one part of the world haven't had time to read all the published papers. There are so many medical journals in existence that a new scientific paper is published every twenty-six seconds. Each month the list of new medical research papers published fills a book that is two inches thick and 1,000 pages long. Computerization does not provide a complete solution to this dilemma.

Our medical libraries are filled with information designed to help doctors help patients. That information lies unused because we put too much emphasis on research and too little on using the information we already have. We spend too much time and effort looking for cures and too little time and effort using the information we already have available. We already know how to prevent eighty per cent of all cancers. And yet doctors still spend most of their time searching for cures for cancer.

The second reason why research programmes are inappropriate is that we need all our healing professionals to put their energies into finding new ways of caring for large numbers of disabled and elderly patients. We can no longer afford to spend time and effort on high-technology diagnostic equipment. We need to spend time and effort on helping people. Many hospitals in Britain are now filled with diagnostic equipment which can detect tumours for which there are as yet no suitable surgical facilities available. This makes a nonsense of a caring profession.

And third, we can no longer care properly for all the sick and disabled who are alive at the moment. And things are going to get much, much worse. If every country in the developed world spent its entire Gross National Product on organ transplantation, there would still be people dying of organ failure. What is the point (or morality) of devising new techniques which we will never be able to make widely available?

COMPUTERS

We need to adopt a far more critical – and imaginative – attitude towards computers and computer technology.

During the last decade many scientists have expressed a tremendous enthusiasm for the power of the computer. In industry, banking, retail outlets, and the home, computer-aided technology has become commonplace. Many experts have expressed the opinion that the next generation of computers – the Japanese call it the fifth generation, the Americans call them 'smart' computers – will be the closest thing to the human brain and will be able to 'think' and 'learn' for themselves.

But before we get too excited by it all it would be wise for us perhaps to ask ourselves whether or not all this is useful progress. It is too easy for us to be taken in by the thought of progress for its own sake so that we forget to ask ourselves whether or not the progress is contributing usefully to our lifestyle or improving our lives in any real way. After all, progress that doesn't improve our lives isn't really progress at all. It is merely scientific advancement. And that is something quite different.

When we take a harsh, critical look at the world of the silicon chip, we find that computers have one very specific weakness. They are stupid.

Computer scientists always do their best to disguise this fact. They claim that computers are logical and able to make decisions far more speedily than human beings. But they confuse logic with intelligence. For the big weakness that computers have is that they can only ever find answers to questions that they have already been asked (or to questions that they have been told to ask themselves). Computers can never think up questions of their own. They are perfectly capable of sorting through all the available existing solutions to a specific problem. But they cannot create entirely new solutions. The computer can multiply and divide but it cannot sinbury. It can multiply and divide because it has been taught how to perform these two functions. But it can't sinbury because it doesn't know what the word means. (I don't either. It's a term I've just invented. But my brain, being human and unlimited by formal thought processes, may well be able to devise some activity that I can call sinburying. The computer has to rely on my eccentric mental activities if it is ever to explore really new territory.)

And until neurophysiologists have worked out just how the human brain works (and despite anything you may have read scientists are as far from that as they are from finding out how to turn marsh-mallows into gold) computer scientists will never be able to reproduce the human brain's unique and precious ability to think creatively.

So, when the chips are down the fifth- or sixth-generation computer will still be limited by the fact that it can only think in computer terms. Despite the claims of the computer scientists a mentally deficient pigeon is more creative than the smartest of 'smart' computers.

Despite all this, in the last few years the computer has been desperately oversold. Computers and their operators are hamstrung by their belief in their own effectiveness. And we've been taken in by their confidence. Computers are useful in many, many ways. For example, they could be used to store and classify research information. But we have been blinded by their apparent omniscience into believing that they can solve more problems and deal with more dilemmas than they are really capable of solving. The fact is – and in some large corporations around the world this is going to be a heretical statement – that computer-operated technology isn't always the best, most economic or even the most efficient way of dealing with a problem. Computers are often inappropriate and counterproductive.

Most important of all, our blind enthusiasm for computers has helped to exacerbate some of the social problems (notably unemployment which as I've shown on p. 185 has a devastating effect on health) which are currently leading us towards the 2020 holocaust.

Let me put all this in perspective with a simple example: the ordinary, common or garden petrol station. At the moment the trend is for the world's largest oil companies to introduce more and more high-technology equipment on to their forecourts. The old fashioned 'service station' was replaced by the self-service forecourt. And today the self-service forecourt is being replaced by what are aptly known as 'ghost' stations. Completely unmanned, these gas stations are equipped with computer-operated pumps which receive the customer's credit card and automatically debit his or her bank account.

Theoretically, these 'ghost' stations may be a good idea as far as the operating oil companies are concerned. But customers don't like them very much. Women don't like stopping at a lonely 'ghost' station and serving themselves. They feel vulnerable and frightened.

215

Drivers who are tired and who have travelled a long distance don't much like them either. They prefer the chance for a chat and the opportunity to buy a soft drink, a bar of chocolate, or a magazine.

So, who, I wonder, is going to be the first highly paid marketing executive to realize that sales of petrol would go up if the human factor were reintroduced? Who is going to be the first marketing 'genius' to realize that if you build a small hut at each 'ghost' station and install a relatively inexpensive station operator then motorists will deliberately aim for that petrol station?

The next step will be for the driver to remain seated in his or her motor car while the operator handles the petrol pump, takes the customer's cash or credit card and operates all the computer machinery too. And the circle will be complete when some enterprising 'ghost' station operator discovers that if he checks customers' oil then he may be able to sell them oil. And that if he offers soft drinks and sweets for sale then he can boost his profits even further. The enterprising individual may even wipe windscreens for tips.

The 'ghost' station is an inappropriate use of computer technology. It is bad for customers (they don't like it). It is bad for petrol station staff (they get made redundant). It is bad for society (more unemployment means more illness and more social-security payments). It is even bad for profits.

The oil industry may yet have some hard lessons to learn. But other industries are already learning. For example, many large and extremely impersonal supermarkets are now introducing delicatessen counters with unwrapped products and personal service. The computer still has a place, of course. You can still pay for your purchase with a credit card. But the limitations of the computer have been recognized.

Controlling the unnecessary spread of computers will lead quite quickly to increased employment, a reduction in stress levels, and a reduction in the amount of disease in our society. By helping to reduce boredom and frustration – the twin threatening consequences of unemployment – we will improve the health of millions.

Some observers will undoubtedly argue that this is a retrograde step – and an impossible one at that. They will say that it is impossible to stop progress. But the criticism, if it comes, will be unjustified.

Computers do have an important place in our society. For example, with a central computer keeping a full list of all hospital consultants and their individual waiting lists the size of Britain's overall waiting list could be halved virtually overnight. Patients in one town destined to wait two years for gall bladder surgery could be taken to a nearby town where the waiting list for the same operation is measured in weeks. The inequalities of the health service could be evened out.

Second, by providing all hospitals and health centres with a computer link-up, we could enable doctors to keep abreast with developments in medicine around the country.

At the moment, if a surgeon in Glasgow develops a new technique it may be months or even years before a surgeon in Brighton hears about the technique. With a properly run computer scheme all doctors could have instant access to a national data bank of information. It wouldn't cost much to run but it would increase the efficiency of the health service enormously.

Third, doctors should be encouraged to use computers to assist them in making diagnoses. Way back in 1974 a team of doctors and computer scientists working in Leeds showed that computers are much better than doctors at making diagnoses. Working with a series of 552 patients a computer had an overall diagnostic accuracy of 91.5 per cent while senior clinicians had an overall diagnostic accuracy of 81.2 per cent. The results of that clinical trial, organized among others by Mr F. T. de Dombal, then Reader in Clinical Information Science at the University Department of Surgery at the General Infirmary in Leeds, were published in the *British Medical Journal* in March 1974. A bigger, later trial, involving 17,000 patients and 250 doctors confirmed that computers are far better than most doctors at diagnosing patients suffering from severe abdominal pains. It was estimated that £23 million of NHS money could be saved by using computers in this way.

By using computers properly we can improve our levels of efficiency and we can improve our health. We can also delay the holocaust I have predicted. At the moment, however, our use of computers is accelerating our progress towards disaster.

MEDIA MEDICINE

Years ago I was commissioned to write a feature about a hospital casualty department for a magazine. It was my intention to write about a typical twenty-four-hour period in the life of a city hospital emergency department.

The day I chose was fairly quiet. There were no major accidents, no major operations and no disasters. In quieter moments of the night the staff confessed that it had been a fairly typical twenty-four-hour period. An examination of the department's record books confirmed this.

But when I wrote my feature an editor at the magazine was

dismayed. 'Where is the blood?' he cried. I protested, pointing out that hospital casualty departments aren't always full of major accident victims. I explained that most of the time the staff have to deal with minor bruises, cuts, poisonings, and drunks. I argued that my article gave a realistic account of life in a hospital casualty department. But the editor wasn't convinced. He wanted blood. And lots of it. He wanted me to go back, wait for a major accident and then write my piece. He couldn't understand when I refused. He couldn't understand why I objected to him attempting to distort the truth and reinforce an inaccurate image. That editor wasn't all that unusual. There is much that is wrong with media medicine today.

Pick up a newspaper and you are still far too likely to find yourself reading about a startling new cure for cancer or arthritis. At the bottom of the news story there will usually be a half-inch paragraph explaining that the cure is as yet only available in Peru or that the initial clinical tests have not yet been started. On the features pages there will be laudatory pieces describing the extraordinary properties of vitamins and minerals and there may be a lengthy profile describing the wonderful work being done by a disabled aromatherapist in Hampstead.

Media medicine is today in the same sort of state that surgery was during the seventeenth century. It is primitive and crude and it almost certainly does far more harm than good. And yet media medicine does have a vital role to play in twentieth- and twenty-first-century medicine. There are three easily definable aspects to that role.

First, and most obvious, it is the role of the media to inform. Twentieth-century patients are brought up to expect far more information than doctors have the time or the training to provide. Patients want facts. They want to know what options are open to them, what alternatives are available, and when to expect signs of improvement.

Patients want to know what they can do themselves, whether they should rest or go to work and whether or not they have to give up sex. They want to know if it is infectious, if there is a vaccine available, and how long they need to take the tablets.

If they don't get the information they need – or feel that they need – then patients worry. If they don't understand the information they are given, then they worry. If they forget what they've been told, then they worry.

Doctors just aren't capable of coping with the enormous thirst for information. They don't have the time to provide explanations in depth and most of them aren't skilled at communicating complicated technical information to untrained, worried individuals. The media's role is to turn incomprehensible technical jargon into easily understandable English.

The second role of the media is to educate the public. Teaching people about health has always been considered important. Back in the days of traditional Greek medicine Hippocrates, the father of medicine, spent much of his time teaching people the importance of eating carefully and exercising regularly. During the Renaissance the remarkable Paracelsus toured the lecture halls of Europe. These days, however, doctors practising orthodox medicine spend very little time teaching patients how to stay healthy or how to deal with minor ailments themselves. When attempts are made to educate people they are usually clumsy, dull, boring, and ineffective.

The final role of media medicine is to watch over new medical developments, to assess the value of new discoveries and new commercial products and to keep a critical watch on all those practising medicine or health care – whether they are orthodox doctors or alternative therapists.

Those are the three theoretical roles of those who work in media medicine. Sadly, those three aims are satisfied far too infrequently.

The first problem lies with doctors themselves. For example, there are those doctors who adore the idea of publicity at any cost. Sometimes the stunts of these publicity-conscious doctors are merely embarrassing. In the last few years there have been numerous occasions when doctors have allowed themselves to be photographed for popular newspapers and magazines. Quite often these vain doctors are responsible for members of the public being exposed to misleading information. A doctor who has performed a modest piece of academic research will boast about his achievement to a journalist and then feign surprise when he finds his name – and details of his work – well publicized.

During the last few years this type of simple vanity has resulted in a good deal of confusion. Doctors who have a strong opinion about something, but who are inexperienced in the ways of the press, will frequently underestimate the power of the media and overestimate the power of their message. It is this type of naive vanity which often leads to medicine being 'oversold', to patients acquiring quite unreasonable expectations, and to the development of a good deal of mistrust between doctors and patients.

Not that doctors seek publicity irresponsibly solely to satisfy their own egos. There are many instances when doctors deliberately seek publicity for straightforward financial motives. The director of a research laboratory who 'leaks' early results which hint at a possible cure for cancer will be hoping that his hand will be

219

strengthened when he applies for his new grant. The drug company medical director who allows his publicity director to issue a press release to journalists is hoping that the reports they write will encourage patients to put pressure on doctors to prescribe his new product.

The second problem lies with the journalists. These can be divided into two main groups. By far the biggest group includes those reporters who do not claim to have any specialist medical knowledge or skills but who are hired to look for news stories and for fresh news angles on old ideas. Journalists in this general category are, by themselves, relatively unlikely to produce articles or programmes which misinform or confuse the public.

Making up a smaller group, but posing a far greater problem, are those journalists who think they know something about medicine. The real problem with some writers is that they think they know everything they need to know. They will have spent some time studying medicine – usually specializing in one particular aspect of health – and will have read a few books and spoken to a few experts. As a result they consider themselves to be specialists. Sadly, they too often provide their readers with inaccurate and misleading advice.

The third problem is produced by the many commercial groups who have a vested interest in manipulating the media and distorting the sort of information which is made available to members of the public. In this category I would put any organization which has an interest in promoting a specific product or type of product.

The result of all this – the vanity of the doctors, the opportunism and ignorance of journalists, the false prophets and the crude commercial requirements of big industry is chaos. Our newspapers are filled with misleading reports, our television screens are full of programmes which distort the facts and bury the truth. And as a result there are millions of confused and bewildered patients and relatives.

If we are to survive into the twenty-first century, then we need those who practise media medicine to uphold a new, strong sense of responsibility. We need journalists who are careful, cautious, and slow to enthuse about new products and new treatments. We need writers and broadcasters who can write about health without distorting the facts, without bowing to commercial prejudices and without ignoring the very real fears, hopes and needs of those who read and listen to their advice.

HIGH TECHNOLOGY

In 1973 the Council for Science and Society was formed with the object of promoting the study of and research into the social effects of science and technology. In 1982 the Council published a report called 'Expensive Medical Techniques'. In that report they concluded that: 'Novel and expensive techniques have been brought into regular use without being evaluated sufficiently, and continued in use when they have become obsolete. Arrangements for systematic clinical trials of new techniques have been haphazard and there has been too little research into their indirect psychological and social effects on patients and their relatives. In many cases the advice of professional committees with very narrow terms of reference has prevailed without consultation of wider expertise and interests.'

Addressing the Thirty-ninth World Health Assembly in 1986 Dr Halfdan Mahler, Director General of the World Health Organization, said: 'One of the main problems is not the lack of appropriate technology, it is the lack of appropriate application of that technology. Even when the will exists to apply it, the best ways of doing so are often not so obvious.'

Looking back over the last few decades it is clear that these criticisms are well founded. Time and time again new treatments such as coronary-artery bypass grafting have been introduced into everyday medical practice without properly conducted clinical trials.

All over the country costly units have been set up and expensive machinery bought on the whim of a surgeon or physician. Hospitals have installed intensive-care units, coronary-care units and heart-transplant teams. And yet these therapies have never been properly assessed. Doctors have spent public money in order to satisfy their personal needs, their professional vanity and their yearning for status and prestige.

New surgical techniques are tried without any attempt to find out whether or not they work. New diagnostic tests are introduced – and widely used – even though no one knows whether or not they work. Psychotherapy is practised by hundreds even though there is no evidence to prove that it does any good at all. New laboratories are built even though there is no justification for their existence. Even when scientific papers are published they are often badly written or poorly designed. One survey reported that out of forty-nine reports on heart surgery there was not one that was properly formulated.

Innovations such as coronary bypass surgery are introduced on a

221

nationwide basis well before trials have been done and before long it is impossible to find a surgeon even prepared to consider that a trial might be necessary.

There are, it seems, no rules. Doctors can behave with arrogance. They can get away with grandiose, heroic schemes for which there is no scientific justification.

We need to decide which treatments work and which are useless. We need to decide which investigations are cost-effective. We need to know which treatments are safe and which are dangerous. We need to assess current methods, established methods and new methods. We need to be critical. We need to be cynical and sceptical. We need to look at the financial and ethical implications. We need to look at running costs and maintenance costs. We need to evaluate patient acceptability. We need to move back towards science and away from superstition. We need to abandon high-technology palliative medicine. We need to introduce controls to stop doctors experimenting with new technologies. We need to assess treatments such as radiotherapy and chemotherapy for cancer – many experts believe that both are used far too often and far too uncritically with the result that many patients suffer unnecessary pain and discomfort.

No new surgical procedures or drug therapies should be introduced without proper testing. We need to be cautious and careful. We need to be rigorous in our attempts to identify worthless surgical procedures and worthless pieces of equipment. We need to encourage criticism and accountability. We need to compare treatments one against the other, and we need to make objective assessments of relative specialities.

Some doctors will undoubtedly claim that too much science in medicine will make treatment less humane. I disagree. *The only humanity in medicine today is a veneer designed to cover up an unscientific approach*. If doctors used science properly, to help provide more knowledge and truth, then humanity would come naturally.

ECONOMICS

The way that the health service is organized does not encourage those who work in it to be conscious of costs. The patient does not pay directly for treatment he receives and there is no insistent reason for doctors, nurses or administrators to concern themselves with costs. The family doctor, for example, has no incentive to economize. He can order whatever tests he wants. He can prescribe whatever he wants (as long as he prescribes drugs from the 'allowed' list). He has such freedom that taxpayers face unlimited liability.

Ironically, while the GP has no incentive to conserve the nation's money he has no incentive to spend his own. A report in October 1986 that was conducted by Nick Bosanquet, senior research fellow, and Brenda Leese, research fellow at York University's Centre for Health Economics, concluded, after studying twenty-five practices in the north of England, that GPs earn more if they spend less on their practice premises and their patients. The GP who puts little back into his practice and has fewer expenses will earn up to fifteen per cent more than the GP who invests money in his practice.

This is all clearly a nonsense. And destructive to the NHS. We need to put some sense back into NHS economics. We need to encourage doctors to put time, effort, energy, and money into their work. And we need to encourage them to save the nation's money by avoiding wasteful practices.

The first step must be to teach those who work in the NHS to understand the principles of health-care economics. Doctors and nurses need to know how budgeting works. Financial accountability should be shown to go hand in hand with professional independence. The best way may be to give individual doctors their own budgets and insist that the limits outlined are rigidly obeyed.

But a wider, public understanding of health-service economics should also be encouraged. Patients and doctors need to understand that not everything is possible – even in the NHS – and that schemes must be considered for cost-effectiveness. One technique may save many lives at a minute cost. Another technique may be so ineffective that it saves only an occasional life for an incredible outlay. It should be clear that it is in the public's interest to choose the first technique and shelve the second.

It is also necessary to compare the costs and the effectiveness of sophisticated treatments. For example, a hip-replacement operation will cost about £750 for each year of 'new life' that it provides. Haemodialysis, on the other hand, costs about £11,000 a year. It isn't fun making comparisons like this, but we all have to accept that there have to be choices in health care. We cannot afford everything. We can no more have everything that is available than the small boy can have everything in Father Christmas' grotto. And yet it is absurd to leave the choices and the decisions about money to specialists who have their own vested interests to support.

Indeed, we need to cut down the amount of money we spend on our hospitals. At present well over two-thirds of the NHS budget goes into the hospital service. And yet only about ten per cent of people who are ill seek any sort of medical advice and only about ten per cent of the people who seek medical advice need the hospital service.

We could save huge amounts of money on heating bills, on administration, on staff, on building maintenance and on equipment by encouraging more surgeons to practice day-case surgery – bringing their patients into hospital for the day only; by insisting that only certain hospitals could ever undertake certain very sophisticated and complicated procedures (reports have shown that there is a much higher success rate when complex procedures are practised at a specialist hospital); and by reopening cottage hospitals where patients, nurses and doctors are all happier and where the costs are much lower.

INCENTIVES FOR DOCTORS

If your doctor is forty years old then he or she is probably dangerously out of date. In the fifteen years or so since qualifying new drugs will have been introduced, new surgical techniques will have been developed and new theories formulated. New diagnostic equipment will have been introduced and old devices abandoned. It is hardly surprising that, in recent years, there has been a dramatic rise in the number of complaints made about general practice and general practitioners.

What is the answer? How can we ensure that doctors keep up to date and remain competent? One of the most popular ideas in official circles at the moment is for the Government to introduce a special awards scheme. The theory is that a group of eminent, leading, carefully selected GPs would sit on a committee and decide which GPs deserve extra money. The hope is that GPs would be encouraged by this incentive to work harder and do their best for their patients. I don't think that such a scheme would help patients at all. All that will happen is that a small, select band of GPs who have the right contacts, the right chums and the right attitude towards authority will find themselves able to afford Rolls-Royces instead of BMWs. It will all be done very secretly and no one will take any account at all of what patients really want from their doctors. I say this with some confidence because there is already an incentive scheme for hospital specialists. And that doesn't work.

The idea behind the Distinction Awards scheme for hospital doctors is that consultants who work unusually hard, who provide patients with a better than average service or who have made some special contribution to medicine will get extra money. On the surface it sounds fair enough. But when you examine what is going on it doesn't look such a good idea.

The first problem is that the Distinction Awards scheme for

hospital consultants is shrouded in secrecy. It is impossible to find out which consultants have been given special awards. I find this difficult to understand. After all, there wouldn't be much point in handing out knighthoods and MBEs if no one knew who had got them.

The second problem is that the evidence does not convince me that the Distinction Awards are given to the right people. Indeed, I believe that awards are given to specialists who know the right people, work in the right hospitals and are members of the right clubs. The facts I've been able to unearth support this contention.

For example, the figures I've obtained for 1986 show that doctors working in London seem to get rather more than their fair share of the loot. The regional breakdown shows that a staggering twenty-eight per cent of awards go to consultants in the London region. These awards, by the way, are not trifling sums. A top award, given on top of a consultant's salary, is £27,300. The figures also show that the people most likely to get awards are not obstetricians, physicians or surgeons but neurosurgeons, neurologists and specialists in nuclear medicine. Are these really the specialists who are most likely to make a valuable contribution to community life?

No, I don't think that an awards scheme for GPs would be a very good idea at all. I think there are a number of far better ways of getting GPs to keep up to date, to do their homework and to do their best to treat their patients well.

Here are just a few schemes which might be suggested if doctors do not deal with these problems themselves. First, patients could be invited to give their doctors marks out of ten for efficiency, courtesy, care, and skill. The marks could then be coordinated nationally (using a computer, of course) and the top GPs given extra bonus payments.

Second, we could introduce an MOT scheme for doctors. Any doctor who is in active practice and who wants to remain on the Medical Register would have to take a requalifying examination every five years or so. The exams would be intended to see whether or not a doctor was keeping up to date. Any doctor failing the exam would have to go back to medical school for a full-time refresher course.

Third, we could start paying doctors by results. We could introduce a scheme whereby doctors only received a payment when they made a positive contribution to a patient's health.

Fourth, there could be a National Inspectorate – like Her Majesty's Inspectorate for Schools. Each practice would be visited every year or two and assessed for efficiency, caring, and competence. Or maybe disguised patients could visit GPs' surgeries – rather like disguised hotel guests visit AA- or RAC-approved hotels. This would enable us to give GPs a rating system.

Fifth, we could have a scheme of punishments. Doctors could be 'fined' if they practised medicine in a slack or lackadaisical way. Doctors could lose ten per cent of their income for keeping patients waiting for routine appointments, for example. Or doctors could lose ten per cent of their income for letting patients collect repeat prescriptions for tranquillizers or sleeping pills.

MEDICAL RECORDS

We would save millions and improve the efficiency of the health service no end simply by allowing patients to keep their own medical records.

If patients kept their medical records with them at home, the records would always be available whether a patient needed to be seen by a GP or a hospital doctor. And this change in administration would enable patients to visit any doctor rather than having to go to the same doctor every time.

The financial savings would come from the fact that thousands of administrators and filing clerks would be released from their onerous duties and would be able to do something useful. Huge amounts of space would be released and the savings on real estate alone would pay for a major, national anti-smoking campaign. And, of course, patients would benefit from the knowledge that their confidential medical information would not be leaked to any outside individual, business or government department.

CARING

In the nineteenth century doctors were long on charity and short on science. Today doctors are long on science and short on charity.

Medicine has gone wrong and needs redirecting. There are serious flaws in the fundamental philosophy followed by most twentieth-century practitioners. Medicine has given society a very costly machine which takes up increasing amounts of money, makes up more and more rules and takes away more and more independence and personal responsibility. There is, today, too little care in assessing new therapies, too little understanding of the real problems. No one seems to bother to ask the fundamental question: 'Will this treatment help this patient live a healthier or longer life? And if so, is that extra life and extra health worth the risk?

Today people are frightened by doctors and the treatments they espouse. Too many therapies are accompanied by unprecedented emotional upheavals. Doctors have become far too obsessed by 'curing' and far too uninterested in 'caring'. While the number of disabled people in our society has risen rapidly, the medical profession has continued to put science first and people second.

Instead of pouring money and resources into providing essential nursing and caring services for the incurable, the disabled and the dying, doctors have spent their time and our money on searches for cures. Fired by personal ambition and professional pride they have spent their time on transplant research, on developing test-tube babies and on searching for new 'wonder' drugs.

In a way this is understandable. It is more exciting to look for a cure than it is to care for the disabled or elderly. Doctors are human and prefer the more dramatic and exciting career prospects. And in a way it makes sense to look for cures. After all, if there were a *cure* for arthritis available then there wouldn't be any need to *care* for patients with arthritis.

But doctors following this fundamental approach have made two fundamental errors. First, they have forgotten that the cures for which they search do not always offer a practicable solution. So, for example, it would never be financially possible to provide heart-transplant operations for everyone needing them. And second, they have gambled too much money and effort on looking for dramatic cures that will help tomorrow's patients with the result that too little effort has gone into caring for today's frail and disabled patients. Indeed, the enthusiasm for curing rather than caring has, with most doctors, become an unhealthy obsession. Medical students are taught nothing about caring and some orthodox doctors seem to feel that anyone who talks about the significance of caring and mental attitudes must be a little odd.

Not surprisingly patients have shown their disappointment and frustration in a number of ways. Most obviously they have turned to others, outside the medical profession, for help. Ironically, many people prefer the caring approach so much that they will turn aside from the curing physician (who may, indeed, have useful treatments available) in favour of the caring quack whose remedies may be even more harmful and less effective than those offered by the physician.

In addition to all this doctors have also ignored the fact that there is now a growing amount of evidence to show that a caring approach can – particularly when applied in conjunction with a potentially useful therapy – produce remarkable results. I dealt with this aspect of healing in some detail on page 181. The fact is that many of the problems which patients take to doctors do not have a physical origin

227

at all but can best be eased by a thoughtful, constructive, caring attitude.

Any doctor who still doubts the real value of a caring attitude should read a paper entitled 'The Effect of a Supportive Companion on Perinatal Problems, Length of Labor and Mother–Infant Inter-reaction' which appeared in the *New England Journal of Medicine*.

The paper showed that when given the support of a lay companion during labour women suffer far fewer complications. Soothed and accompanied women took 8.8 hours to deliver (as opposed to 19.3 hours for unaccompanied women), they were awake more after delivery, they talked to their babies more, and smiled at them more. The authors reported that 'there may be major perinatal benefits of constant human support during labor'.

THE DISABLED

As I have already shown, the size of Britain's disabled population is going to grow dramatically during the next few years. If the problems produced by that expanding population of disabled individuals are not going to overwhelm us, then we need to act now.

First, discrimination against the disabled should be curbed. In 1986 the Spastics Society conducted a survey of London employers which showed that disabled people applying for jobs still face blatant discrimination. A researcher working for the Spastics Society sent two letters of application in fictitious, English-sounding names to each of 157 employers who had advertised for secretaries. One of the letters appeared to come from an able-bodied woman, the other from a woman of the same age, status and experience but with cerebral palsy. Of the able-bodied applicants ninety-seven per cent were sent application forms, asked to attend an interview or telephoned for more information. But only fifty-six per cent of the disabled applicants were invited to attend interviews, sent application forms or telephoned. Forty-one per cent of the employers turned down the disabled applicant straightaway. In some cases the disabled applicant was told that the job was filled while the able-bodied applicant was invited to an interview.

This sort of discrimination will inevitably lead to frustration and anger among the disabled and, paradoxically, to resentment among the able-bodied who will object to the fact that the disabled always live on social-security benefits.

Second, money needs to be spent altering patients' homes so that they can look after themselves outside a hospital environment. There should also be more money spent on district-nursing services.

Homes need to be converted so that accommodation can be provided on the ground floor only. Or better, wider, more accessible lifts need to be installed. Research needs doing to find the best ways of helping disabled patients and money needs spending to experiment with new techniques and new aids.

Third, money should be spent getting rid of steps and building ramps in towns and cities. Many local authorities have already spent some money on making public places more accessible for patients in wheelchairs or patients who are disabled in other ways. But the facilities available are still far too patchy and cannot be relied upon.

Fourth, sheltered accommodation needs building for disabled and elderly people. Some sheltered accommodation has already been built. But nowhere near enough. Unemployment is one of the major problems in our society. There is plenty of work here to keep millions of people employed. The work will not run out. And the money will be available if we cut back our expenditure on unnecessary and wasteful high-technology medicine.

SPECIALIZATION

As high-technology medicine has become more and more important so more and more specialities have developed. The growth of specialization over the last twenty years or so has been stimulated by doctors themselves rather than by the needs of patients. Today there are well over a hundred different specialities and within each speciality there are numerous 'superspecialists' who have dedicated their professional lives to the study of minutiae. As specialists become better and better at less and less, it is difficult to avoid the disturbing conclusion that they will eventually be superb at doing absolutely nothing.

The more doctors specialize the more removed they become from the real problems of everyday medical practice. Specialists tend to spend a good deal of their time on esoteric research projects; they consider their patients as research fodder rather than as individuals in need of support, help or care.

Modern specialists design their working day not around the requirements of their patients, but around the capabilities of the equipment at their disposal. The equipment is not there to help them heal their patients; the patients are there to help them use the equipment. Doctors order the equipment they use so subsequently they have to justify the expense by making use of it as much as possible.

There are numerous dangers and disadvantages in it all for

patients. To begin with the type of treatment a patient receives will depend upon the type of specialist he sees. If you go to a gastroenterologist with a stomach pain, you'll have your stomach X-rayed. If you go to a gynaecologist with a stomach pain, you'll have your uterus and ovaries examined. If you go to a psychiatrist with stomach pain, you'll be talked to and asked about your sex life. If you go to an orthopaedic surgeon with stomach pain, you'll have your back looked at. If you go to a neurologist with stomach pain, your nervous system will be checked out. If you go to a gland specialist with stomach pain, then your glands will get an overhaul. If you go to a cardiologist with stomach pain, then you'll have heart tests. If you go to an acupuncturist then you'll get treated with needles. If you go to a herbalist, then you'll get herbs. And so on and so on. If you go to a car dealer who sells Ford motor cars, then he'll sell you a Ford. If you go to a brain surgeon with a pain, he'll probably operate on your brain. It's as simple as that.

The whole sorry business is made far, far worse by the fact that the majority of specialists think of themselves as 'superior' beings. They consider themselves to be the most important part of the system. They treat patients arrogantly and rudely. They humiliate patients. They subject them to unnecessary tests and examinations. They *use* them.

Specialists insist on their patients coming into hospital to suit their personal habits. And then they let patients go home according to their own personal whims. So, for example, if a surgeon plays golf on a Friday and doesn't come into the hospital at the weekend, then a patient who could have gone home on Friday morning will stay there until Monday morning. No junior doctor will dare to discharge a patient without his senior's permission.

If patients want to refuse treatment, they have to sign a form which suggests that they are lunatics who don't know what they are doing. If patients want to know what is going on or ask questions, they will be considered a nuisance and a troublemaker. Doctors don't like troublemakers (although, paradoxically, troublemakers live longer and survive hospitals better – research has shown that more aggressive patients are far more likely to live to tell the tale of their hospital stay).

And yet despite all this apparent authority, conceit and arrogance specialists are not, by and large, particularly good at what they do. Specialists aren't usually much better than GPs at making diagnoses. They make the same sort of mistakes, and their knowledge of drugs is equally rudimentary.

To all this must be added the fact that specialists, being narrow-minded and fixated on one area of health, are frequently likely to treat a non-existent problem or to treat a problem that doesn't matter while ignoring a problem that does matter.

Too often the only difference between a specialist and a GP is that a specialist makes erroneous decisions with more certainty. Specialists are convinced of their own infallibility and it is, sadly, their patients who suffer as a result.

I believe that a number of the problems within the NHS could be conquered if the number of specialists around was reduced and their power and authority drastically reduced. In some cases whole specialities could easily disappear. There is, for example, no justification for specialists in the treatment of the elderly (geriatrics) or specialists in the treatment of the mind (psychiatry). In neither case is there any genuine, technical need for doctors to specialize in these areas. By and large old people suffer from the same illnesses as middle-aged people. And psychiatry is largely myth not science.

In other cases specialists should merely be demoted to a more sensible role. The radiologist is simply a technician who reads X-ray plates. The anaesthetist is merely a technician who puts people to sleep. The surgeon is merely a plumber who operates on faulty bodies. We need technicians to carry out operations, perform diagnostic tests and look after patients who do need hospital care.

I can see no justification for allowing specialists to retain financial control over huge departments, nor for allowing them to retain control over other technicians working within the hospital environment. Specialists do not understand social implications, budgetary control and, most important of all, the peculiar needs of the individual patient.

The training that specialists receive, the rewards they enjoy and the power they exercise are all excessive. We would move towards 2020 in a far more healthy state if specialists working in hospitals were considered to be nothing more nor less than technicians who offer patients a specific service.

EUTHANASIA

When Aristotle Onassis died in 1975 his doctors boasted that he had been dead three times before they finally let him go. When Spain's Franco was trying to die he had to fight a team of thirty-two doctors who were determined to keep him alive. Franco had twenty different diseases but he was kept 'alive' in a coma for thirty-four days. He was sedated, he had tubes in every orifice, he was on a kidney machine, he was helped to breathe by a machine, he had a defibrillator permanently strapped to his chest, he had a tube in his stomach, he had a pump to keep his blood flowing around his body, he received a total of 120 pints of blood by transfusion (in other words he had his blood supply replaced twelve times) and he suffered endlessly. Before he finally lapsed into his coma he is reported to have had a lot of pain. But his doctors didn't dare give him painkillers because they would have interfered with the life-saving processes that had been started.

Sadly, doctors have been encouraged to strive to preserve the sanctity of life at all costs. Terrified of lawsuits and professional disciplinary committees doctors struggle to keep their patients alive even when there is no longer any real life or living to protect.

Pneumonia used to be called the 'old man's friend' since it often offered the elderly a peaceful and dignified death. Today too few people are allowed to die in peace or dignity. Doctors have put the healing emphasis on the treatment of conditions which threaten life rather than on conditions which disable. It is hardly surprising that the number of seventy- and eighty-year-olds in our society is rising. Nor that the number of disabled seventy- or eighty-year-olds is rising. The sad but controversial truth is that too few octogenarians die of pneumonia these days.

It isn't just doctors who are responsible for this attitude, of course. Social workers and relatives are responsible too – fired often by a potent mixture of guilt, shame and embarrassment. When I practised medicine a few years ago I often found myself pressured by young relatives and social workers who wanted old people put back into hospital. The old people frequently wanted to stay at home. The argument put forward by the social workers and young relatives was that if he were left alone, Grandad might fall and break a leg or might set fire to himself. Grandad was invariably happy to take that risk. He didn't mind dying. He preferred the risk of dying contentedly at home to the inevitability of dying without dignity in hospital. But the social workers and the young relatives couldn't cope with the responsibility. I confess that I frequently overruled them and allowed old people to live – or die – at home. There is far less danger or terror in the average terraced house than in the average hospital. But many doctors would disagree with me. They would side with the social workers. They would refuse to accept the responsibility.

But the real problem is that once patients get into hospital they may be injured by machines and doctors, they may be damaged and tortured by tests and investigations, but they won't be allowed to die. They will certainly not be allowed to die of anything as simple as old age or pneumonia. We have created such wonderful ways of keeping people alive artificially that we now have to create artificial ways to let people die. Instead of a peaceful, natural death we have created a society in which extremists talk about euthanasia and 'mercy killing'. Instead of the gentle sleep we think of pills and injections and suffocation. Is it any wonder that increasing numbers of old people kill themselves these days? Too often suicide is the only way out for them.

I believe that doctors have no right to strive officiously to keep elderly patients alive against their will. I think that patients who are old and tired and weak and weary are entitled to a natural, peaceful death. I don't think we need legislation or rules or moral arguments to help us solve this problem. I think we need nothing more complicated than love and care. Sometimes the most loving thing a doctor or relative can do is to let a patient die.

MEDICAL SCHOOLS

Patients have enormous faith in doctors. They do what they say. They trust them in a way that they would never trust or obey plumbers, electricians, accountants or lawyers. Their trust may be built out of fear but it is, nevertheless, trust. But too many doctors are not worthy of that trust.

Too many doctors are rude, arrogant, patronizing, paternalistic and contemptuous. Doctors leap on new ideas with regrettable enthusiasm. They consider themselves infallible when they are only too fallible. They specialize in lucrative practices. They waste time and money (usually someone else's). They look after one another, they cling together, they protect and preserve the secrecy of the profession. They perform unnecessary operations. They take authority but deny responsibility. They insist on having power over social events like birth and death where, in truth, they have no role. The most powerful weapon against death is the will to live but most doctors weaken this weapon by their daily practices. They continually fail to nurture the patient's own self healing skills.

Too often doctors ignore patients with chronic diseases; the very patients who most need caring and compassion. They ignore diseases which do not carry kudos or satisfy their professional ambitions.

Too often doctors treat the disease not the man. They fail to see a man's illness within the framework of his life. They forget that the man may be frightened about money, death, illness, unemployment or loneliness. They do not seem to understand that the majority of diseases could be cured by a holiday or a football pool win. They look always for a physical explanation where one doesn't always exist.

Doctors base their assessments and conclusions on assumptions, prejudices, hearsay, subjective observations, personal interpretations and the conclusions of colleagues who may or may not be right. Doctors are too often narrowminded and too often they allow their personal experiences and interpretations to control their thinking. A few years ago every surgeon 'knew' that the best treatment for breast cancer was a radical mastectomy. And there are still thousands of doctors performing this crude, destructive and unforgivable operation. Worthless, dangerous treatments are practised without any scientific basis or humanitarian justification. Doctors are blinkered and fixated too; the surgeon who operates on varicose veins assumes that the world is full of people suffering from varicose veins. He does not see the myriad other problems which cause so much devastation.

Doctors treat their patients like objects. They get no marks for courtesy or kindness. They withhold information from their patients. They part with facts as if they were pearls. They use medical terminology to build up barriers. They wear white coats to build up barriers. They emphasize every difference they can find between human beings and doctors, and never fail to exhibit their power. They consider that their responsibilities are not to patients but to other doctors; to one another. They do not seem to understand the feelings, the fears and the anxieties of their patients. They are technicians lost in a world where there should be compassion but there is only curiosity.

Too often doctors overprescribe, overinvestigate and overtreat. They don't listen, don't understand and don't seem to care. According to Dr Mahler, the thoughtful and sensitive Director General of the World Health Organization, 'the major and most expensive part of medical knowledge as applied today appears to be more for the satisfaction of the health professions than for the benefit of the consumers of health care'.

Medicine today is for the doctors not the patients. Home deliveries have gone for pregnant women. Home visiting has been reduced to a minimum. Family doctors rely on duty rostas and deputizing services. Cottage hospitals are closed. Battery hospitals have replaced them.

Doctors practise defensive medicine. They close ranks in self-protection. Is it any wonder that millions turn to alternative medicine for support and help?

Doctors claim to be scientists. But they are not scientists. Doctors who use scientific tools are no more scientists than typists who use word processors are computer specialists. In medicine the application of science is very unscientific. In true science ideas are born and tested before conclusions are drawn; in medicine there is no testing.

Ideas are obtained from drug-company representatives or other commercial advisors. The true scientist excludes probability, chance and coincidence. The doctor has too much pride, too much vanity, too large an ego for such deference to science.

Doctors learn and practise by pronouncement. There is no questioning, no doubting, no thought.

Doctors prefer mystique and authority to impartial knowledge. They will draw conclusions from a single case history published in a medical journal or from a single personal experience. They will make predictions and choose remedies as a result of prejudices which may well be wildly inaccurate. They allow themselves to distort information to obtain a conclusion they want.

Doctors operate on the principle of normal values. They will treat any patient whose blood tests show a variation from the considered 'norm' – even though there is no such thing as 'normal'; even though the patient may be perfectly well. In modern medicine laboratory values are like religious principles.

The fundamental deception in modern medicine is that doctors have special healing powers. Doctors do not understand that the technology they use in order to treat their patients can be harmful when applied improperly.

Modern medicine is not so much a science as a superstition. Doctors treat themselves or the lesion rather than the patient. They treat abnormalities not distress. Their success is measured in the laboratory not in the bed.

Because they don't like subjecting their ideas to the risk of failure, doctors do not often test their theories. They prefer to practise. Patients may suffer through their professional vanity.

Several thousand years ago doctors believed that patients were made ill by the anger of the gods. They believed that cures were effected when the anger was appeased. Today doctors do not worship gods, but they worship equally primitive remedies. They worship drugs and surgery and high-technology equipment. They worship cardiac angiography and electrocardiography. The modern god is not disembodied. He has a plug on the end of him. He is fired not by the spirit of the universe but by electricity.

The modern doctor is obsessed with interventionism. It is this constant need to interfere that is one of the sources of the profession's inadequacies and limitations. Doctors rely on instruments with which to dignify their intervention. They explain *their* success by pointing to drugs and surgical equipment. A few thousand years ago they would have pointed with equal conviction to herbs, songs, dances, rattles, chants, special ceremonial incantations and handfuls of bones thrown on to the dust. There is no more sense in

235

one than in the other. The handful of bones are as scientific as the Electroconvulsive Therapy machine.

Doctors have presence, authority and power. They have status in the home, and can violate normal physical and social taboos. They expect, and are given, respect. They expect gratitude and trust from their patients. These emotional attitudes are built out of experience but based on fear and a need to find someone in this uncertain world to trust. Doctors tend to believe that these rights are theirs automatically. They believe that they have exclusive healing rights over their patients. They become proprietorial. They do not like their patients to be educated. All these attitudes, all these faults, all these errors of understanding are all produced deliberately within the medical school.

The foundation of modern medical thinking is the Cartesian principle that the body and the mind can be treated separately. Modern medical training is still based on the philosophies of Descartes who believed in mechanical man. The modern clinician is taught to base opinions and conclusions on observations and experience but not taught to question those observations. Nor is he encouraged to see the mind and the body as a single unit. Holistic principles are alien to the newly trained medical graduate. Doctors excuse their reluctance to test their observations by claiming that to do so would be to deprive patients of help.

Today we no longer need high-technology medicine. We no longer need doctors who are dedicated to curing. We no longer need doctors who are devoted to the principles of interventionism. There is no role for orthodox, traditional medicine of this type.

Patients want caring doctors. The biggest problem of the twenty-first century will be to care for the elderly and the disabled. We now need compassion and dignity. We need doctors who recognize that there is no treatment for the sadness of bereavement other than comfort and support. We need doctors who can encourage us to show love and affection because those are the remedies we have available. We need to utilize our natural resources because we can no longer afford to subsidize the unnatural resources so honoured by doctors.

If doctors are to have a major role in the twenty-first century, medical schools will have to change and to change rapidly. There will have to be a change of emphasis from disease to people. Students will have to be trained to understand that the environment is everything. The hospital is an unnatural place; little or no training should take place there.

For years the training of doctors has been unsuited to the needs of the patients. There is now a crisis of confidence and understanding. Patients are beginning to turn elsewhere for help – to homoeopaths, acupuncturists, herbalists, and gurus of all kinds. They are turning to new religions, or to drugs; anything that offers hope or escape. One or the other.

I have already explained that I believe that in the future the role of the specialist will have to be reconsidered and downgraded. In the twenty-first century the only real role for doctors will be in general practice. But there doctors must fit in to the needs of the patient or else they will have no future.

Doctors have to break away from the Cartesian dogma. They have to accept that the shortcomings associated with our health system can only be conquered by a medical revolution. We need a broader system of health care in which illness is seen as a result of an interaction between mind, body and environment. We need to stop thinking of illness as a mechanical breakdown which can be repaired in a mechanical, superficial way.

We can deal with the cost and ineffectiveness of our health system. We can deal with our current excess of doctors by persuading some to work in developing countries. We can overcome the problems offered by high technology.

But if the medical profession is going to have a genuine part to play in helping us avoid the holocaust of 2020 then doctors – and medical schools – are going to have to change their whole philosophy of life. Today medicine is about curing not caring. Medicine isn't about keeping people healthy. It is about pseudo-science. It is something that Galen and Paracelsus would have understood.

It is too late for that now. We do not need that sort of medicine any more. We need something much simpler.

AND . . .

All this will help. But it will not, of course, be enough.

We must take a much tougher line with companies selling products which damage health. We have to increase taxes on tobacco and alcohol by several thousand per cent. They have to be priced out of business. We have to bring in controls to ensure that the distribution of high fat products such as butter and cream is minimalized and not promoted. We have to control drug-marketing programmes. There is no time for half-hearted measures. We must be tough.

Individually, none of these answers will solve our problems permanently. But if we do all these things now, if we make the changes that I have recommended, then we will be able to delay the time when the percentage of sick and disabled individuals in our society exceeds the percentage of healthy individuals. We will give ourselves a breathing space in which we can look for other solutions, other answers, other possibilities.

If we do not make all these changes now, then before the twenty-first century is two decades old the human race will have moved irretrievably towards the point of no return and we will have ensured our own eventual destruction.

INDEX

241

strokes, 8, 90, 200–1
suicide, 4, 91–2, 93, 105, 203, 233
sulphonamides, 18
Summerlin, Dr William, 111
Surgam, 34
surgery, 61–8; breast replacement, 89;
    iatrogenesis, 46; psychosurgery,
    93–6; waiting lists, 6, 61, 126, 142,
    147–53, 216–17; wasteful practices,
    133–4
Sutherland, Ian, 166
Sykes, P. A., 149
syphilis, 76

Talbot, Dr Ian, 53
tamoxifen, 90
Taylor, Dr Brent, 5
Taylor, George, 72–3
technology, 69–90, 161, 163–75, 221–2
TENS machines, 36–8, 146
tests and investigations, 73–8, 85–6,
    127–9
tetracyclines, 51–2, 132
Thames Television, 13
Thomas, Dr K. B., 181–2
Thompson, John, 36–7
The Times, 23
tobacco industry, 24–6, 165, 166
tonsillectomy, 61, 62, 63
Townsend, Peter, 183–4
tranquillizers, 103–8
transplant operations, 155, 157–60
Trattler, Ross, 197–8
Treasury, 165
tuberculosis, 19
TV AM, 23

unemployment, 185–6, 216
United States Bureau of the Census, 7
University of California Medical
    Center, 80
University College Hospital, London,
    146
Update, 6, 22, 49–50, 66, 86, 96, 123,
    186

vaccination, whooping-cough, 17–20
Valium, 103, 104
varicose veins, 197
Veronesi, Dr Umberto, 67
Vessey, Martin, 175
Veterans' Administration Hospitals,
    65, 80, 105
vivisection, 115

waiting lists, 61, 126, 142, 147–53,
    216–17
Wall, Dr John, 51
Walton Hospital, Liverpool, 128
Warneford Hospital, Oxford, 66
Waterson, M. J., 30
Way, Dr Lawrence, 80
welfare state, 203–5
Wellcome, 15
Welsby, Dr Philip, 13
Whalley, Neil, 133
Whitney, Ray, 140
whooping-cough vaccine, 17–20
Wigley, Margaret, 118, 119
Wills, Mr, 69–71
Withington Hospital, Manchester, 146
Wood, Dr Clive, 23
Woodland, Dr Richard, 120
World Health, 46
World Health Assembly, 26–7, 221
World Health Forum, 170, 171–2
World Health Organization (WHO),
    22, 25–6, 27, 41, 46–7, 78, 95, 112,
    114, 131, 167–8

X-rays, 77–8, 79, 110, 128, 129, 173–4

Yale School of Medicine, 112
Yale University, 45
Yates, John, 150

Zilbergeld, Bernie, 101
Zola, Emile, 163
Zomax, 53